**Virtual Patient Encounters**

# Implementation Manual

*for*

Sanders:

Mosby's Paramedic Textbook

Revised Third Edition

# Virtual Patient Encounters
# Implementation Manual
*for*

Sanders:
Mosby's Paramedic Textbook
Revised Third Edition

*Implementation Manual prepared by*
**Kim D. McKenna, RN, BSN, CEN, EMT-P**
Director of Education
St. Charles County Ambulance District
St. Peters, Missouri

Software developed by
**Wolfsong Informatics, LLC**
Tucson, Arizona

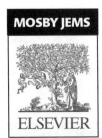

# MOSBY JEMS
### ELSEVIER

11830 Westline Industrial Drive
St. Louis, Missouri 63146

VIRTUAL PATIENT ENCOUNTERS IMPLEMENTATION MANUAL     ISBN: 978-0-323-04936-8
FOR SANDERS: MOSBY'S PARAMEDIC TEXTBOOK
REVISED THIRD EDITION

---

### Notice

Knowledge and best practice in this field are constantly changing. As new research and experience broaden our knowledge, changes in practice, treatment and drug therapy may become necessary or appropriate. Readers are advised to check the most current information provided (i) on procedures featured or (ii) by the manufacturer of each product to be administered, to verify the recommended dose or formula, the method and duration of administration, and contraindications. It is the responsibility of the practitioner, relying on their own experience and knowledge of the patient, to make diagnoses, to determine dosages and the best treatment for each individual patient, and to take all appropriate safety precautions. To the fullest extent of the law, neither the Publisher nor the Author assumes any liability for any injury and/or damage to persons or property arising out or related to any use of the material contained in this book.

---

ISBN: 978-0-323-04936-8

*Publishing Director:* Andrew Allen
*Executive Editor:* Linda Honeycutt
*Managing Editor:* Scott Weaver
*Publishing Services Manager:* Linda McKinley
*Senior Project Manager:* Kelly E.M. Steinmann
*Cover Designer:* Mark Oberkrom

Printed in United States of America

Last digit is the print number: 9 8 7 6 5 4 3 2 1

# Contents

*Summative lesson—see "Introduction—To the Instructor" for an explanation.

*Summative lesson—see "Introduction—To the Instructor" for an explanation.

# Summative Lessons Listed by Case

Case 1: 20-year-old male—difficulty breathing (Lesson 28)

Case 2: 56-year-old female—fell (Lesson 23)

Case 3: 7-year-old female—seizure (Lesson 26)

Case 4: 64-year-old male—unknown medical (Lesson 27)

Case 5: 40-year-old male—vomiting blood (Lesson 29)

Case 6: 16-year-old female—unknown medical (Lesson 31)

Case 7: 8-year-old male—submersion (Lesson 39)

Case 8: 38-year-old male—suicide attempt (Lesson 35)

Case 9: 22-year-old female—assault (Lesson 42)

Case 10: 25-year-old female—abdominal pain (Lesson 37)

Case 11: 32-year-old male—gunshot wounds (Lesson 21)

Case 12: 57-year-old male—man down (Lesson 33)

Case 13: 5-month-old male—unresponsive (Lesson 40)

Case 14: 65-year-old male—difficulty breathing (Lesson 24)

Case 15: 42-year-old male—difficulty breathing (Lesson 25)

# Acknowledgments

Virtual Patient Encounters was developed over the past 3 years with input from many emergency medical services (EMS) instructors around the United States, who participated in some fashion or another. Some traveled across the country to share their vision of what a valuable critical-thinking product would be; others wrote cases and recommended management sequences; some provided their expertise at focus groups and user-centered design studies; and many, many instructors reviewed the software, study guide, and implementation manual.

We are deeply grateful to each of you for helping us make this implementation manual a reality. Your education, dedication, and experience clearly shine through in this one-of-a-kind educational product for paramedic students everywhere. Recognizing your contributions wherever you were involved—in the software, the study guide, and/or the implementation manual does not truly express our gratitude.

I would like to offer a very special thank you to three of the best instructors in EMS who worked tirelessly creating this product and graciously made the many changes recommended by other subject matter experts: Twink Dalton, whose creative juices were never-ending; John Gosford, whose field experience and technical expertise brought road-ready reality into each case. You two were a dynamic duo. Your shining lights were bright even on the dreariest of days, and your energy and enthusiasm were contagious. A special thank you is also extended to Kim McKenna, who thought it would be so much fun to write the study guide and implementation manual. Your determination to see this project through its completion, even when the task was arduous and seemed overwhelming, delivered a finished product that is nothing short of genius. We are deeply indebted to each of you and owe you a large replacement supply of midnight oil.

To paramedic instructors: I hope Virtual Patient Encounters fills in the frustrating gap of trying to prepare students to be critical thinkers and make the right clinical decisions for their patients before they enter their clinical experiences and the field.

Finally, to Scott Weaver: Your eye for detail, as well as your patience and perseverance, have paid off. You are now an honorary paramedic, in spite of your challenges with pharmacology. Can you say vacation?

*Linda Honeycutt*
*Executive Editor*

# Implementation Manual Reviewers

**Jane Bedford,** RN, CCEMT-P
Chief Training Officer
Nature Coast EMS
Inverness, Florida

**Jon Cooper,** NREMT-P
Lieutenant
Baltimore City Fire and EMS Academy
Baltimore, Maryland

**John A. DeArmond,** NREMT-P
Director
Emergency Management Resources
Half Moon Bay, California

**Steven Dralle,** LP, EMSC
General Manager
American Medical Response, South Division
San Antonio, Texas

**Dennis Edgerly,** EMT-P
Paramedic Education Coordinator
HealthONE EMS
Englewood, Colorado

**Janet Fitts,** RN, BSN, CEN, TNS, EMT-P
Educational Consultant
Prehospital Emergency Medical Education
Pacific, Missouri

**Rudy Garrett,** AS, NREMT-P, CCEMT-P
Flight Paramedic
Lifenet Aeromedical Services
Somerset, Kentucky

**Mark Goldstein,** RN, BSN, EMT-P I/C
EMS Coordinator
William Beaumont Hospital
Royal Oak, Michigan
Adjunct EMS Faculty
Oakland Community College
Auburn Hills, Michigan

**John Gosford,** BS, EMT-P
Associate Professor and EMS Coordinator
Lake City Community College
Lake City, Florida

**Leslie Hernandez,** BS, NREMT-P
Advanced Program Director
Bulverde-Spring Branch EMS
Spring Branch, Texas

**Scott C. Holliday,** BS, EMT-P
Deputy Chief of EMS Training
FDNY
New York, New York

**Larry Richmond,** AS, NREMT-P, CCEMT-P
EMS Education Manager
Mountain Plains Health Consortium
Ft. Meade, South Dakota

**Robert Vroman,** BS NREMT-P
EMS Instructor
HealthONE EMS
Englewood, Colorado

# Introduction—To the Instructor

Virtual Patient Encounters (VPE) is designed to complement *Mosby's Paramedic Textbook, Revised Third Edition*. This combination of textbook, study guide, and simulation software creates a unique "learning triad" that enables your students to apply what they are learning in a unique hands-on way, thereby developing essential clinical decision-making skills. Drawing upon 15 challenging emergency cases in the software, the study guide provokes the student to think critically and begin bridging the gap between book knowledge and street smarts.

This implementation manual was created specifically to help you, the instructor, integrate VPE into your classroom. We recommend that you carefully read the following sections before beginning to use VPE with your students:

- **Preparing for Virtual Patient Encounters** provides an overview of all the information you need to implement VPE into your teaching, including tips for preparing yourself and your classroom. Most important, this section suggests ways to prepare your students so they know what is expected of them.

- **Getting Started** provides all the information you need to install VPE, set up the program, and adjust your computer settings.

- **Orientation to Virtual Patient Encounters** serves as a comprehensive review of all the functionality in the simulation software. (This section is also included in your students' study guide.)

- **Optional Online Resources** serves as a guide to using the Evolve Learning System, a comprehensive and flexible online learning system that provides you and your students with a structured method for delivering course content via the Internet. In this section you will find complete instructions for requesting VPE resources on Evolve and enrolling your students in the unique course you have created.

After you have read these sections, you will find another section entitled **"Implementing Virtual Patient Encounters,"** which recommends student assignments and relevant review topics, as well as suggested class activities and discussion questions for each lesson found in the student study guide. Also included are suggested answers to each lesson's exercises.

Since Virtual Patient Encounters is intended to promote critical thinking, students should complete a number of "prerequisites" before attempting each study guide lesson, including reading their assignment from *Mosby's Paramedic Textbook* and completing any skills, laboratory studies, and pertinent activities from the *Workbook for Mosby's Paramedic Textbook*. You should also review the most relevant topics with your students before they complete each lesson; a bulleted "Topic Review" list is provided for this purpose.

It is envisioned that each student will complete the study guide lessons as homework, either using their home computer or the school's computer laboratory. During the next class you may want to review the assignment and allow the students to lead the discussion on what should be done to manage the patient and why, which will provide you with additional insight into your students' abilities to think critically and to make correct clinical decisions. As a "follow-up" to each lesson, this implementation manual also provides some suggested ideas for in-class activities and questions to have students answer as a group. Make sure your students are given an opportunity to express any problems or questions they have. Remember, the cases in VPE offer a unique opportunity for all your students to experience and discuss the same clinical experience—something that rarely, if ever, happens on their incident runs.

If you would like, you can also assess your students using the test bank questions found in the Evolve Learning System. See "Optional Online Resources" on page xli for more information on this and other online features of VPE.

**Using the VPE Study Guide with Your Students.** The lessons in your students' study guide follow the same order as the table of contents in the textbook. However, as with chapters in the textbook, it is not necessary to assign them in that order. For example, Lesson 14: Assessment-Based Management, asks students to read Chapters 14, 25, 29, 33, 36, 38, and 40 before completing the lesson because some of the exercises require students to develop an action plan. Consequently, you may wish to assign Lesson 14 after the students have "mastered" all of the previously mentioned chapters. Another example is Lesson 24: Cardiology II, which has some exercises that address respiratory issues. If you follow the order of the textbook, "Pulmonology" follows "Cardiology." You may wish to assign this lesson after completing the chapter on "Pulmonology."

In general, the lessons in the student study guide can be divided into two categories—"foundational" and "summative" lessons. Foundational lessons are primarily concentrated on the early chapters in the textbook when students are learning preparatory content. The focus of these lessons is building foundational knowledge. Many of these chapters entail accessing and comparing multiple cases on the software but without actually attempting to care for the patient just yet.

Summative lessons require a broader understanding of many concepts from different chapters before being attempted. These are marked with an asterisk in the table of contents. It is highly recommended that your students read the specific chapter in the reading assignment, as well as all the chapters listed as "relevant," before attempting these summative lessons.

**Intentional errors.** Be aware that deliberate "errors" are planted in the simulated cases to set up exercises in the study guide, particularly in the videos. For example, in the video of the suicidal patient in Case 8, the police have hog-tied the patient and placed him face down on the stretcher. Several lessons prod the student to describe how this situation should be rectified. Other elements may be present in the cases with which you, yourself, disagree: use this disagreement to your advantage and bring it up as a class discussion. Critiquing the performance of the EMS personnel in the videos can be a powerful learning tool.

**Variations in vital signs.** The simulated patients in the Virtual Patient Encounters software respond to interventions performed by students. Just as in real life, if students repeat certain assessments consecutively on the simulated patients, some vital signs (e.g., blood pressure, pulse, and respiratory rate when patient is tachypneic) may vary by slightly above or below the previous reading. These variations are considered insignificant and do not reflect any intervention or decision on the student's part.

**Recommended sequences of care.** The appendix at the end of this implementation manual includes 15 tables—one for each case in the software. Each table lists the sequence of care for each case consistent with *Mosby's Paramedic Textbook* and the 1998 National Standard Curriculum for the EMT-Paramedic and as recommended by our panels of subject-matter experts. The software is programmed to deliver the best results if each sequence of interventions is followed for each case.

Other sequences may result in acceptable outcomes as well. As in "real" life, poor care will result in poor patient outcomes. Of course, treatment protocols vary by locale; consequently, these recommended sequences should not be considered "absolute." For this reason the software does not automatically "grade" the student's performance; rather, it provides a complete log of every assessment and intervention the student performs so that you, the instructor, can evaluate it.

All the summative lessons will direct your students to care for the relevant case from beginning to end and then answer the exercises in the study guide while consulting their log. At the end of each summative lesson is a "Summary Activity" in which students are asked to critique their own performance and then compare it with the recommended sequence in consultation with you. This is your opportunity to provide individualized feedback on the students' critical-thinking skills as revealed by the combination of their log from the software and their answers to the study guide exercises. If you want students to turn in their logs, they can do so by either printing it out from the software and handing in a hard copy or by saving it as a rich-text file and e-mailing it to you.

We hope this implementation manual helps you successfully incorporate Virtual Patient Encounters into your paramedic program.

# Preparing for Virtual Patient Encounters

## PREPARING YOURSELF

In the front of the student Study Guide (and also included in this Implementation Manual beginning on page xix) are **Getting Started** and **Orientation** sections that explain the installation and navigation of Virtual Patient Encounters. Please read these sections to familiarize yourself with the software and how it functions.

### Software Notes

- Please be sure your system is compatible with the VPE software by checking the system requirements on page xix of this Implementation Manual.
- Insert the VPE program disk into your CD-ROM drive and follow the step-by-step instructions given in the **Getting Started** section beginning on page xix of this Implementation Manual.
- Please take a few moments to become familiar with the software so that you have a better understanding of how it functions.
- The **Optional Online Resources** section of this Implementation Manual will give you the necessary information for accessing the Virtual Patient Encounters online resources through the Evolve website.

## PREPARING YOUR CLASSROOM

If you plan to use the software and/or the Evolve website (see the **Optional Online Resources** section in this manual) in your classroom, you will need the following items:

- Projector screen
- Computer that meets the system requirements
- Mouse
- External speakers so that the videos can be heard in the classroom
- LCD projector
- VPE program disk
- PowerPoint slides

When preparing to use the VPE software or the Evolve site in class, it is always a good idea to set up the room before the start of class so that you do not have to waste valuable class time preparing.

Install the VPE program disk or access the Evolve website before the start of class so that you are ready when class begins.

If using the PowerPoint slides provided, install the slides on the classroom computer or bring the disk to class with you. *Note:* You can also print the slides and give them as handouts to students for taking notes.

### Viewing and Printing PowerPoint Slides in Notes Pages Format

Before the start of class, you can open and print the PowerPoint slides in Notes Pages format. Once the file is open, select **Print** from the File menu or simply click on the Print icon on the tool bar near the top of the screen. Then change the print format from Slides to Notes Pages in the drop-down menu near the lower-left corner of the Print menu before clicking **OK**.

## PREPARING YOUR STUDENTS

The first step in orienting your students to VPE is to require them to read the **Getting Started** and **Orientation** sections of their Study Guide. This experience will help relieve any anxiety they may have about using an interactive software program such as VPE. This is especially true for nontraditional students who may not be comfortable with computers.

Explain the benefits of VPE to your students.

- Serves as a clinical primer to ease their transition into clinical experiences and the field.
- Stimulates critical thinking skills.
- Helps prepare them for certification testing.
- Provides hands-on learning.
- Reinforces the importance of following established protocols.

Point out the system requirements located on the back cover of the student study guide. Explain that using the software on a system that does not meet the requirements can cause problems and malfunctions with the software.

Point out the following available resources:

- **Getting Started** section in the front of the study guide
- **Orientation** section in the front of the study guide
- Evolve website (see **Optional Online Resources** section of this manual)

## GUIDELINES FOR IMPLEMENTING VPE

1. **Start Out Slowly**

   Remember that there is a learning curve for you and your students. Ease students into the software until you have a feel for how well they are progressing. As they become more familiar with how VPE works and the time it takes to complete assignments, you will be able to increase the number of lessons/activities you assign. *Note: VPE is not intended to be a grading or testing tool. It is designed to complement your existing classroom resources and help students improve their overall test scores.*

## 2. Be Time-Sensitive

Make a note of the time estimation provided next to each exercise in the study guide so that you know how much time outside of class students will be spending. In the beginning, exercises may take longer to complete since students are still learning to navigate the software. Many of the lessons were created to be fully completed in one classroom period or within a manageable time frame if given as a take-home assignment. However, most lessons are composed of several smaller exercises that can be completed individually should students need to stop and finish the lesson at a later time.

## 3. Remind Students Not to Procrastinate with Assignments

When assigning lessons/exercises, always remind students not to procrastinate! This may seem like obvious advice, but it is especially important with VPE assignments because of the potential for unexpected delays that can occur when using computer-based components, particularly when using the **Online Study Guide**. If students wait too long to begin an assignment and then encounter an unexpected problem—for instance, their computer "crashes" or their Internet server goes down—they may be unable to complete the assignment on time.

# Getting Started

## ■ Getting Set Up

### SYSTEM REQUIREMENTS

#### WINDOWS™

- Windows® PC
- Windows XP
- Pentium® processor (or equivalent) @ 1 GHz (2 GHz or greater is recommended)
- 1.5 GB hard disk space
- 512 MB of RAM (1 GB or more is recommended)
- CD-ROM drive
- 800 × 600 screen size
- Thousands of colors
- Soundblaster 16 soundcard compatibility
- Stereo speakers or headphones

#### MACINTOSH®

Virtual Patient Encounters is not compatible with the Macintosh platform.

### INSTALLATION INSTRUCTIONS

#### WINDOWS™

1. Insert the Virtual Patient Encounters CD-ROM.
2. Inserting the CD should automatically bring up the set-up screen if the current product is not already installed.
    a. If the set-up screen does not automatically appear (and Virtual Patient Encounters has not been already installed), navigate to the **My Computer** icon on your desktop or in your **Start** menu.

---

Trademarks: Windows, Pentium, and America Online are registered trademarks.

    b. Double-click on your CD-ROM drive.

    c. If installation does not start at this point:

        (1) Click the **Start** icon on the task bar, and select the **Run** option.

        (2) Type d:\setup.exe (where "d:\" is your CD-ROM drive), and press **OK**.

        (3) Follow the onscreen instructions for installation.

3. Follow the onscreen instructions during the set-up process.

## HOW TO LAUNCH VIRTUAL PATIENT ENCOUNTERS

### WINDOWS™

1. Double-click on the **Virtual Patient Encounters ALS** icon located on your desktop.

2. **(alternative)** Navigate to the program via the Windows **Start** menu.

## SCREEN SETTINGS

For best results, your computer monitor resolution should be set at a minimum of $800 \times 600$. The number of colors displayed should be set to "thousands or higher" (High Color or 16-bit) or "millions of colors" (True Color or 24-bit).

### WINDOWS™

1. From the Start menu, select **Settings**, then **Control Panel**.

2. Double-click on the **Display** icon.

3. Click on the **Settings** tab.

4. Under **Screen Resolution**, use the slider bar to select **$800 \times 600$ pixels**.

5. Access the **Colors** drop-down menu by clicking on the down arrow.

6. Select **High Color (16-bit)** or **True Color (24-bit)**.

7. Click on **OK**.

8. You may be asked to verify the setting changes. Click **Yes**.

9. You may be asked to restart your computer to accept the changes. Click **Yes**.

## TECHNICAL SUPPORT

Technical support for this product is available between 7:30 AM and 7:00 PM (CST), Monday through Friday. Before calling, be sure your computer meets the recommended system requirements to run this software. Inside the United States and Canada, call 1-800-692-9010. Outside North America, call 1-314-872-8370. You may also fax your questions to 1-314-523-4932, or contact Technical Support through e-mail: technical.support@elsevier.com.

## ■ Virtual Patient Encounters Online Study Guide

To use the *Virtual Patient Encounters Online Study Guide,* you will need access to a computer that is connected to the Internet and equipped with web browser software that supports frames. For optimal performance, speakers and a high-speed Internet connection are recommended. However, slower dial-up modems (56 K minimum) are acceptable.

## WEB BROWSERS

Supported web browsers include Microsoft Internet Explorer (IE), version 6.0 or higher; Netscape, version 7.1 or higher; and Mozilla Firefox, version 1.5 or higher.

If you use America Online (AOL) for web access, you will need AOL, version 4.0 or higher, and IE, version 5.0 or higher. Do not use earlier versions of AOL with earlier versions of IE because you will have difficulty accessing many features.

For best results with AOL:

- Connect to the Internet using AOL, version 4.0 or higher.
- Open a private chat in AOL (this allows the AOL client to remain open without asking whether you wish to disconnect while minimized).
- Minimize AOL.
- Launch a recommended browser.

Whichever browser you use, the browser preferences must be set to enable cookies and JavaScript, and the cache must be set to reload every time.

### ENABLE COOKIES

| Browser | Steps |
|---|---|
| Internet Explorer (IE), version 6.0 or higher | 1. Select **Tools** → **Internet Options**.<br>2. Select **Privacy** tab.<br>3. Use the slider (slide down) to **Accept All Cookies**.<br>4. Click **OK**.<br><br>**OR**<br><br>3. Click the **Advanced** button.<br>4. Click the checkbox next to **Override Automatic Cookie Handling**.<br>5. Click the **Accept** radio buttons under **First-Party Cookies and Third-Party Cookies**.<br>6. Click **OK**. |
| Netscape, version 7.1 or higher | 1. Select **Edit** → **Preferences**<br>2. Select **Privacy & Security**.<br>3. Select **Cookies**.<br>4. Select **Enable All Cookies**. |
| Mozilla Firefox, version 1.5 or higher | 1. Select **Tools** → **Internet Options**.<br>2. Select the **Privacy** icon.<br>3. Click to expand **Cookies**.<br>4. Select **Allow** sites to set cookies.<br>5. Click **OK**. |

### ENABLE JAVASCRIPT

| Browser | Steps |
|---|---|
| Internet Explorer (IE), version 6.0 or higher | 1. Select **Tools** → **Internet Options**.<br>2. Select **Security** tab.<br>3. Under **Security** level for this zone, set to **Medium** or lower. |

| Browser | Steps |
|---|---|
| Netscape, version 7.1 or higher | 1. Select **Edit → Preferences**<br>2. Select **Advanced**.<br>3. Select **Scripts & Plugins**.<br>4. Make sure the **Navigator** box is checked to **Enable JavaScript**.<br>5. Click **OK**. |
| Mozilla Firefox, version 1.5 or higher | 1. Select **Tools → Options**.<br>2. Select the **Content** icon.<br>3. Select **Enable JavaScript**.<br>4. Click **OK**. |

### SET CACHE TO ALWAYS RELOAD A PAGE

| Browser | Steps |
|---|---|
| Internet Explorer (IE), version 6.0 or higher | 1. Select **Tools → Internet Options**.<br>2. Select **General** tab.<br>3. Go to the **Temporary Internet Files**, and click the **Settings** button.<br>4. Select the radio button for **Every visit to the page**, and click **OK** when complete. |
| Netscape, version 7.1 or higher | 1. Select **Edit → Preferences**<br>2. Select **Advanced**.<br>3. Select **Cache**.<br>4. Select the **Every time I view the page** radio button.<br>5. Click **OK**. |
| Mozilla Firefox, version 1.5 or higher | 1. **Select Tools → Options**.<br>2. Select the **Privacy** icon.<br>3. Click to expand **Cache**.<br>4. Set the value to "**0**" in the **Use up to: ___ MB of disk space for the cache** field.<br>5. Click **OK**. |

## PLUG-INS

 **Adobe Acrobat Reader**—With the free Acrobat Reader software, you can view and print Adobe PDFs. Many Evolve products offer student and instructor manuals, checklists, and more in the PDF format!
**Download at:** http://www.adobe.com

 **Apple QuickTime**—Install this software to hear word pronunciations, heart and lung sounds, and many other helpful audio clips in the Evolve Online Courses!
**Download at:** http://www.apple.com

**Adobe Flash Player**—This player will enhance your viewing of many Evolve web pages, as well as educational short- to long-form animation in the Evolve Learning System!
**Download at:** http://www.adobe.com

 **Adobe Shockwave Player**—Shockwave is best for viewing the many interactive learning activities in Evolve Online Courses!
**Download at:** http://www.adobe.com

 **Microsoft Word Viewer**—With this viewer, Microsoft Word users can share documents with those who do not have Word, and users without Word can open and view Word documents. Many Evolve products have test banks, student and instructor manuals, and other documents available for downloading and viewing on your own computer!
**Download at:** http://www.microsoft.com

 **Microsoft PowerPoint Viewer**—View PowerPoint 97, 2000, and 2002 presentations with this viewer, even if you do not have PowerPoint. Many Evolve products have slides available for downloading and viewing on your own computer!
**Download at:** http://www.microsoft.com

## SUPPORT INFORMATION

Live support is available to customers in the United States and Canada from 7:30 AM to 7:00 PM (CST), Monday through Friday, by calling **1-800-401-9962**. You can also send an e-mail to evolve-support@elsevier.com.

In addition, **24/7 support information** is available on the Evolve web site (http://evolve.elsevier.com) including:

- Guided tours
- Tutorials
- Frequently asked questions (FAQs)
- Online copies of course user guides
- And much more!

# Orientation to Virtual Patient Encounters

Welcome to Virtual Patient Encounters!

The course of study to become a paramedic is complex and involves not only a narrow look at a specific topic, but being a paramedic also requires that you have a broad foundation of knowledge from which to pull to enable you to provide effective and safe patient care. Sometimes discrimination among similar choices is required. In the textbooks, patient presentation offers only a clear, one-faceted look at each illness or injury. When reading, patient care may seem similarly straightforward and the path to the correct decisions and interventions may appear very clear. In contrast, real patient situations are often fuzzy, complex, and confusing. This combination of study guide with simulation software is designed to help you bridge the gap between the books and the street and to assist you in "putting it all together." We hope you will reflect on the knowledge from each of the foundation chapters when you evaluate and treat these patients. It is our goal that this course of study will make your transition to the field easier and will give you the confidence to make the right decisions when they matter the most.

## BEFORE YOU START

For best results, use the Virtual Patient Encounters simulation software as directed by the lessons found in this study guide. Each lesson begins with a reading assignment, usually a single chapter in your textbook. Make sure to read this material before beginning the lesson because you will need to understand the concepts before attempting to answer the questions in the study guide or before you make any patient care decisions in the software. Some lessons also list "relevant" chapters in addition to the reading assignment. These *summative* lessons will require a broad understanding of many concepts from different topic areas before being attempted. We highly recommend that you read all these relevant chapters in addition to the reading assignment before attempting the summative lessons.

The following icons are used throughout the study guide to help you quickly identify particular activities and assignments:

**Reading Assignment**—Tells you which textbook chapter(s) you should read before starting each lesson.

**Writing Activity**—Certain activities focus on written responses such as filling out forms or completing documentation.

 **CD-ROM Activity**—Marks the beginning of an activity that uses the Virtual Patient Encounters simulation software.

 **Reference**—Indicates questions and activities that require you to consult your textbook.

 **Time**—Indicates the approximate amount of time needed to complete the exercise.

Each lesson in the study guide provides specific directions that explain what to do in the software to prepare for each exercise. These directions are always bulleted and are always indicated by an arrow (→) in the left margin. Do no more or no less than what the directions indicate. For example, many lessons require that you watch only a video before answering the study guide questions, whereas others will direct you to also perform your initial assessment in the software. Summative lessons will direct you to care for the patient from beginning to end as best you can, based on what you have learned from the textbook and in class.

Although the study guide lessons provide specific directions as to what to do in the software, when it comes to caring for the patients (e.g., performing assessments and interventions), you will need to understand what all the buttons do. The following orientation will explain the entire software interface and how you can treat each of the 15 cases.

## HOW TO LOG IN

To open the Virtual Patient Encounters simulation program, you can either double click the Virtual Patient Encounters ALS icon that should appear on your computer desktop after you have installed the software, or you can click on **Start**, then **Programs**, then **Virtual Patient Encounters**, then **Virtual Patient Encounters ALS**. Once the program begins, you will see an anti-piracy warning and a video montage before the log-on screen appears (shown below). If you wish to skip the video montage, click on the **Skip Intro** button at the bottom of the screen.

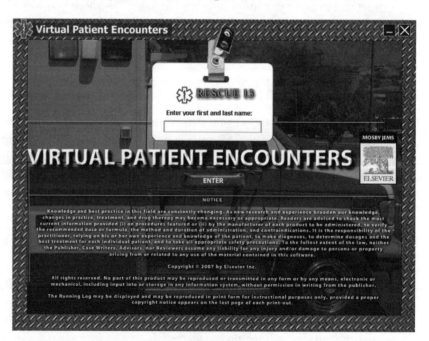

Type your first and last names into the name tag pictured, and click **Enter**. This will take you to a list of all 15 cases in this program (shown in the first screen on the following page).

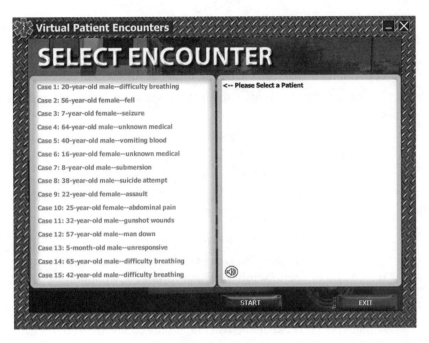

Once you click on a patient, you can listen to the dispatch report, which will also appear as text in the panel on the right side of the screen. (If you don't want to hear the dispatch audio, you can click on the **MUTE** icon.) After you have listened to and read the dispatch information, you can then click **START** to respond to the case. (An **EXIT** button also appears on this screen if you want to close the entire program.)

Once you select a case, your initial approach to the scene and patient will play in a video. All the videos include an overview of the area from the perspective of the ambulance (shown below) to enable you to think about staging considerations and scene safety.

On approaching the patient, you will have an opportunity to perform the scene size-up, form an initial visual impression of the patient, and listen to information provided by conscious patients and any first responders, family members, or bystanders on the scene. Be aware that

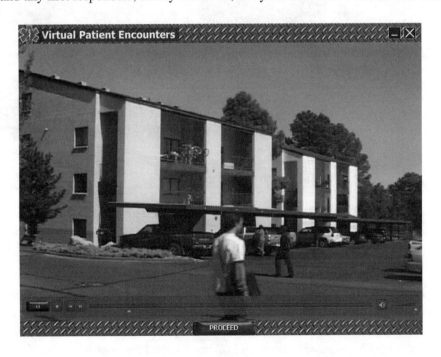

some videos intentionally deviate from "best practice" to give you a chance to critique how things were handled. In addition, interventions, such as spinal immobilization, which would have been performed immediately in some cases, were not shown in the video to give you the opportunity to make all the decisions about patient care once the video concludes.

The video controls are similar to those found in many popular media players. Here is what each one does:

❚❚ (Pause)—Pauses or "freezes" the video on the current frame.

▶ **PLAY**—Resumes playing the video from the point where it has been paused or from the beginning if the video has been stopped.

■ **STOP**—Stops the video entirely. To restart the video, you must click **PLAY** (▶).

◀◀ **REWIND**—Restarts the video from the beginning.

▶▶ **FORWARD**—Jumps several frames forward in the video.

Two slider bars are also provided. The long slider bar across most of the width of the screen allows you to scroll back and forth to any point in the video. Simply double click and hold the triangle (▲), then drag it to the left to go to an earlier moment or to the right to go to a later moment. The short slider bar on the far right controls the volume of the video's audio. A mute button between the two slider bars can be clicked to turn off the audio altogether.

When the video reaches the end, it automatically will forward you to the patient care interface, which is described below. If you want to skip the video altogether and go directly to the patient care interface, you can click on the **PROCEED** button at the bottom of the video screen.

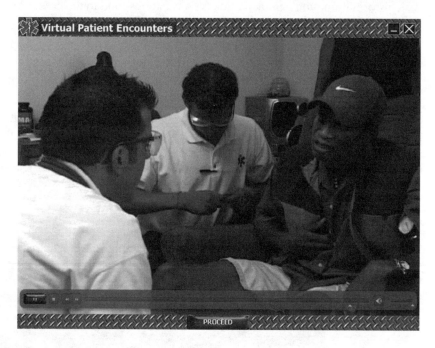

## PATIENT CARE INTERFACE

The patient care interface consists of three panels: (1) Patient Care Panel, (2) Patient Visual Panel, and (3) Running Log as described in the following text.

### Patient Care Panel

The Patient Care Panel runs along the left side of the screen and consists primarily of two distinct areas (shown at the top of the following page): (1) contains all the controls for performing assessments and (2) contains all the controls for performing interventions.

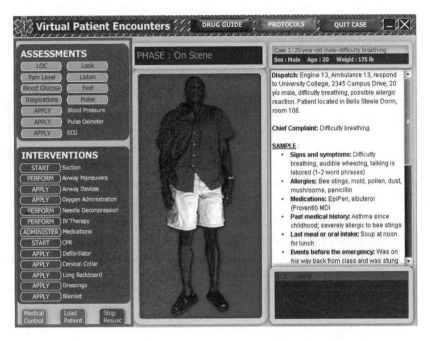

## ASSESSMENT CONTROLS

The assessment controls allow you to gather information on each patient so you can decide which interventions would be appropriate to care for him or her. These control buttons allow you to perform your patient assessments. Each button is described individually.

**LOC** (Level of Consciousness)—Click the **LOC** button to reveal the patient's current level of consciousness in the running log on the right side of the screen. In some cases the patient's orientation will be below the level of consciousness if it is pertinent to the case. Be aware that the patient's level of consciousness may change, depending on what interventions you perform. For instance, administering a sedative may decrease the patient's level of consciousness.

**Pain Level**—Click the **Pain Level** button to reveal the patient's current pain level on the 1-to-10 scale. The patient's pain level can increase or decrease, depending on your treatment; for example, administering a narcotic to a patient with a high pain level may decrease his or her level of pain.

**Blood Glucose**—Click the **Blood Glucose** button to reveal the patient's current blood glucose reading. Treatments such as administering 50% dextrose could affect this reading.

**Respirations**—Click the **Respirations** button to reveal the patient's current respiratory rate and quality. The respiration rate and quality can also be affected by your patient care decisions. For example, the patient's respiratory rate will slow after administering midazolam.

**Pulse**—Click the **Pulse** button to reveal the patient's current pulse rate, regularity, and strength. Your patient care decisions can affect these three measurements. For example, administering atropine sulfate will slow the patient's heart rate.

**Blood Pressure**—Click the **APPLY** button for blood pressure to place a blood pressure cuff on the patient and to receive your first reading. Once the cuff is on the patient, you only need to click the **READ** button that appears to the right for subsequent readings. If you want to remove the blood pressure cuff, you can click the **REMOVE** button that replaces the **APPLY** button. Interventions such as dopamine administration can affect blood pressure.

**Pulse Oximeter**—Click the **APPLY** button for pulse oximeter to place a finger clip on the patient and to receive your first oxygen saturation (SaO$_2$) reading. Once the clip is on the patient, you only need to click the **READ** button that appears to the right for subsequent readings. If you want to remove the finger clip, you can click the **REMOVE** button that replaces the **APPLY** button. Interventions such as administering oxygen to the patient in respiratory distress can affect $SaO_2$ readings.

**ECG**—Click the **APPLY** button next to the ECG button to place leads on the patient and display a dynamic ECG tracing on the monitor in the lower right corner of the screen, immediately below the running log. Note that this ECG is a 3-lead ECG and that lead II is being displayed. Twelve-lead ECGs for several cases are included in the relevant study guide lessons for your evaluation. If you want to remove the ECG, you can click the **REMOVE** button that replaces the **APPLY** button. Make sure to keep your eyes on the ECG tracing because it can change unexpectedly or in response to your treatment decisions.

**Look**—Click the **Look** button to open a "wizard" that allows you to receive visual information about the patient's head and neck, chest and abdomen, upper extremities, lower extremities, back, and genitalia. Simply click on the body area you want to know about, and then click **ASSESS**. (Click **CANCEL** if you want to exit the wizard.) The following information is displayed in the running log for each body area:

*Head and Neck*
- Pupil size*
- Pupil reactivity*
- Skin color*
- Mouth*
- Nose*
- Other observations
- DCAP-BTLS

*Chest and Abdomen*
- Check excursion*
- Skin color*
- Other observations
- DCAP-BTLS

*Upper Extremities*
- Skin color*
- Other observations
- DCAP-BTLS

*Lower Extremities*
- Skin color*
- Other observations
- DCAP-BTLS

*Back*
- Skin color*
- Other observations
- DCAP-BTLS

*Genitalia*
- Other observations
- DCAP-BTLS

The above items with an asterisk may change in response to your treatment decisions; do not forget to reassess often.

**Listen**—Click the **Listen** button to open a wizard that allows you to receive aural information about the patient's heart and lungs. Simply click on the organ you want to know about, and then click **ASSESS**. (Click **CANCEL** if you want to exit the wizard.) The following information is displayed in the running log for each:

*Heart*
- Heart rate*
- Heart regularity*

*Lungs*
- Left lung sounds*
- Right lung sounds*

The above items with an asterisk may change in response to your treatment decisions; do not forget to reassess often.

**Feel**—Click the **Feel** button to open a wizard that allows you to receive tactile information about the patient's head and neck, chest and abdomen, upper extremities, lower extremities, and back. Simply click on the body area you want to know about and then click **ASSESS**. (Click **CANCEL** if you want to exit the wizard.) The following information is displayed in the running log for each body area:

*Head and Neck*
- Skin temperature*
- Skin moisture*
- Other observations
- DCAP-BTLS

*Chest and Abdomen*
- Skin temperature*
- Skin moisture*
- Other observations
- DCAP-BTLS

*Upper Extremities*
- Skin temperature*
- Skin moisture*
- Other observations
- DCAP-BTLS

*Lower Extremities*
- Skin temperature*
- Skin moisture*
- Other observations
- DCAP-BTLS

*Back*
- Skin temperature*
- Skin moisture*
- Other observations
- DCAP-BTLS

The above items with an asterisk may change in response to your treatment decisions; do not forget to reassess often.

### INTERVENTION CONTROLS

The intervention buttons will allow you to treat each patient in accordance with what you have learned in your textbook and in class, as well as what you think are the issues with each patient based on information you have gathered from the opening video, the patient's history, and any assessments you have performed. Each intervention that you perform may cause realistic changes in the patient, which you can determine by conducting ongoing assessments. Each intervention button is described individually below.

**Suction**—Click **START** to clear the patient's airway. Click **STOP** to end suctioning.

**Airway Maneuvers**—Click **PERFORM** to open a wizard that will allow you to choose to perform an abdominal thrust, a head-tilt/chin-lift, or a jaw thrust. Simply click on the maneuver you would like to perform.

**Airway Devices**—Click **APPLY** to open a wizard that will allow you to choose from the following airway devices:

- Oropharyngeal airway
- Nasopharyngeal airway
- Endotracheal tube
- Laryngeal mask
- Cricothyrotomy
- Combitube

If you select the endotracheal tube, you will be prompted to select multiple methods for confirming the correct tube placement. Click **REMOVE** to remove the airway device currently in use.

**Oxygen Administration**—Click **APPLY** to open a wizard that will allow you select from the following types of oxygen and ventilation devices:

- Nasal cannula
- Simple face mask
- Partial rebreather mask
- Nonrebreather mask
- Bag-mask at 12 breaths/min
- Bag-mask at 20 breaths/min

Once you select one of the above devices, you will be prompted to select an oxygen flow rate. Click **REMOVE** to remove the type of oxygen or ventilation device currently in use.

**Needle Decompression**—Click **PERFORM** to open a wizard that will allow you to select a needle gauge before performing needle decompression. Because needle decompression is an intervention that cannot be undone, the program will not permit you to perform this intervention on any patient for whom it would be inappropriate.

**IV Therapy**—Click **PERFORM** to open a wizard that will allow you to start an intravenous (IV) or intraosseous line for medication administration or fluid therapy.

Five steps to this wizard are listed as follows:

1. Select whether you want to start a left or right peripheral IV or get intraosseous access (shown at the top of the following page). Click **NEXT** after you have made your choice (or **CANCEL** to close the wizard altogether).

2. Select which type of fluid you want to infuse. Click **NEXT** after you have made your choice (or **BACK** to return to the previous step or **CANCEL** to close the wizard altogether).

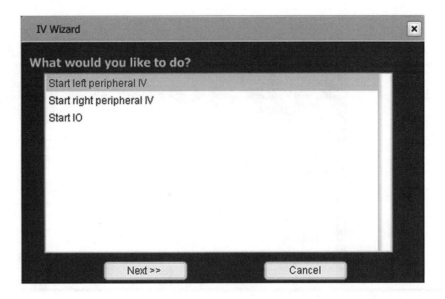

3. Select the rate of infusion you want: select either TKO (To Keep Open) to provide a route for administering medications or Wide Open for fluid replacement therapy. Wide Open can also be used to administer medications intravenously in addition to fluid therapy. Click **NEXT** after you have made your choice (or **BACK** to return to the previous step or **CANCEL** to close the wizard altogether).

4. If you chose TKO on the third step, the next step allows you to select your catheter size and tubing. If you chose Wide Open on the third step, you have to select your fluid amount before you select your catheter size and tubing. Always click **NEXT** to advance to the next step, **BACK** to return to the previous step, or **CANCEL** to close the wizard altogether.

5. The last step allows you to confirm all your selections before committing to them. Read over what you selected; if your selections are what you want, then click **DONE**. If you want to make modifications, click **BACK** to return to the step where you want to make changes. Make your changes, and click **NEXT** until you get back to the confirmation step. As always, clicking the **CANCEL** button will close the wizard without any effect on the patient.

Once you have started an IV or intraosseous line, you can reopen the IV Therapy wizard again and again by clicking **PERFORM**. When you reopen the wizard, you will see a slightly different set of options at the first step. You can choose one of the following:

1. Start another line,

2. Remove a line that you have already started, or

3. Administer additional fluids to any of the lines you already started.

Use the **NEXT, BACK**, and **DONE** buttons to make and confirm your selections.

You will also notice that a **FLUSH** button appears in the panel to the right once you have started a line. You can click on this button and flush any of the lines that you have already started.

**Medications**—Click **ADMINISTER** to open a wizard that allows you to administer medications to the patient.

The wizard has four steps:

1. Select the medication you want to administer from the alphabetical list of generic drug names displayed (see figure on the following page). You can review the list of medications using the scroll bar on the right side of the wizard. If you want to look up more information about a drug, click the **Drug Guide** button. This button will open

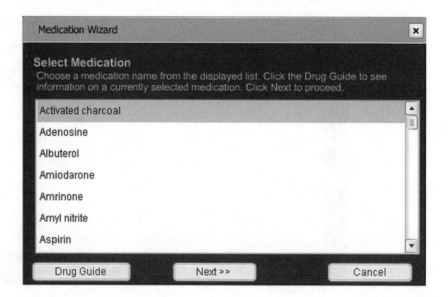

a searchable resource that will be described in greater detail later in this orientation session. Highlight the medication you want to administer by clicking on its name, and then click **NEXT**. (Click **CANCEL** to exit the wizard altogether.)

2. Select the route you want to use to administer the drug you selected in the first step. Again, you can review the list of routes using the scroll bar on the right. (Note that the IV and intraosseous routes will not appear on this list unless you have already started them using the IV Therapy wizard as previously described. If you need to administer a drug using one of these routes, click **CANCEL** to close the medication wizard and then open the IV Therapy wizard to start a line first. Then you can reopen the medication wizard, and you will now find the route listed at the second step.) Highlight the route you want to use, and then click **NEXT**. (Click **CANCEL** to exit the wizard altogether.) If you select an incorrect route for the drug you selected at the first step, you will receive a message to that effect and be instructed to click **BACK** and make a different route selection. Be aware that your incorrect route selection will be recorded on the running log, so make your selections carefully.

3. Select the dose you want to administer of the drug you selected in the first step. Be aware that each dose may have a different effect on the patient. Highlight the dose you want to administer, and then click **NEXT**. (Click **CANCEL** to exit the wizard altogether.)

4. The last step allows you to confirm all your selections before committing to them. Read over what you selected; if all selections are what you want, then click **FINISH**. If you want to make modifications, click **BACK** to return to the step where you want to make changes. Make your changes, and click **NEXT** until you get back to the confirmation step. As always, **CANCEL** will close the wizard without any effect on the patient. Note that if you select the IV or intraosseous route at the second step, you will have to select whether you want to inject the medication as an IV push or IV infusion before you can confirm your selections. You must select an IV type that is compatible with the medication and dose you selected earlier to proceed. If you make the wrong selection, your mistake will be recorded in the running log.

**CPR**—Click **START** to begin performing cardiopulmonary resuscitation (CPR) on the patient. Click **STOP** to stop CPR.

**Defibrillator**—Click **APPLY** to place defibrillator pads on the patient. Click **REMOVE** to remove the pads. To defibrillate the patient, click on the **PACE/SHOCK** button that appears in the panel to the right. This selection will open a wizard; you must first select whether you want to start pacing or to shock the patient in either sync or unsync mode. If you start pacing the patient, you have to reopen this wizard to stop pacing. If you choose to shock the patient in either sync or unsync mode, you will then be prompted to select an energy level. When you click on an energy level, the shock will be delivered to the patient. You can also click **BACK** to return to the initial screen or **CANCEL** to close the wizard without any effects on the patient.

**IMPORTANT:** Be aware that the defibrillator simulated in the software is intended to be used as a monophasic machine. A monophasic defibrillator was simulated instead of a biphasic machine because recommended energy levels are consistent from manufacturer to manufacturer, whereas energy levels for biphasic machines currently vary, depending on the make of the machine. Although biphasic defibrillators have become very common, monophasic machines are still in use and may be encountered both in the classroom and in the field. Keep this in mind when selecting which energy level to administer when using the defibrillator.

**Cervical Collar**—Click **APPLY** to place a cervical collar on the patient. Click **REMOVE** to remove it.

**Long Backboard**—Click **APPLY** to place the patient on a long backboard. Click **REMOVE** to remove it.

**Dressings**—Click **APPLY** to place dressings on any wounds the patient may have. (Nothing will happen if the patient does not have wounds.) Click **REMOVE** to remove the dressings.

**Blanket**—Click **APPLY** to place a blanket on the patient. Click **REMOVE** to remove the blanket.

### "OTHER" BUTTONS

Three additional buttons below the intervention controls level are available for use during patient care:

**Medical Control**—Click the **Medical Control** button if you want to contact medical control. In this program you can contact medical control to request additional orders or to request permission to stop resuscitation. Consult medical control if you are having trouble figuring out which protocol(s) to follow for a particular case. They will eventually point you in the right direction. They will give you permission to stop resuscitation only if resuscitating the patient is not possible.

**Stop Resusc**—If medical control gives you permission to stop resuscitation, you may click the **Stop Rescusc** button. If you click the **Stop Resusc** button, you will be asked to confirm your decision. If you click *yes* to confirm, stopping resuscitation will be recorded in your log. Keep in mind that if you stop resuscitation without requesting permission from medical control or if permission was denied, all of this will be recorded in your log for your instructor to evaluate.

**Load/Unload Patient**—When you first enter the patient care interface, you are considered to be "on scene." While on scene this button will display as **Load Patient**. Click this button when you believe transporting the patient is most appropriate. Your decision to load will be recorded in the running log in the context of all your assessments and interventions. Once you have loaded the patient, you are considered to be in transit and this button changes to display as **Unload Patient**.

You may have noticed that time is not counted in this program. Although this is a luxury you will not have in real life, removing the time element allows you to think about your decisions before you make them, rather than simply trying to "beat the clock," particularly because assessments and interventions are not done in real time. Virtual Patient Encounters is not intended to be used as a game.

Although the study guide may pose situations in which you have limited time in transit and asks questions about how you would adjust your treatment, in the software program you can continue performing interventions and assessments while in transit for as long as you believe you can make a difference. Once there is nothing more you can do besides provide support and monitor your patient, then you can click **UNLOAD PATIENT**.

## Patient Visual Panel

The panel in the middle of the interface displays the patient in the supine position from a top-down perspective (shown below).

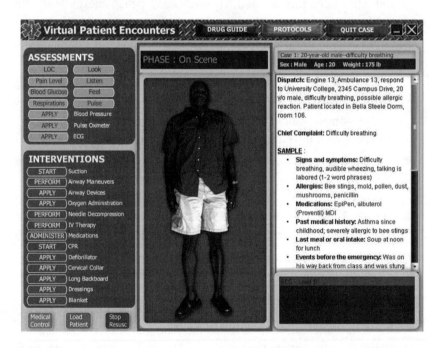

As you perform your assessments and interventions, the equipment you use appears on the patient in this panel. For example, when you click **APPLY Blood Pressure**, a blood pressure cuff will appear on the patient's arm; and when you click **APPLY Oxygen Administration** and select a nonrebreather mask, an image of a nonrebreather mask will appear on the patient; and so on. The patient visual panel is intended to give you a visual indication of what equipment is currently in use on the patient. The equipment images are representative of real equipment but may not always appear exactly as they would in real life; for example, when a long backboard is used, the patient would be secured to it with straps and a head immobilization device.

When you start CPR using the intervention buttons, you will see a pair of hands repeatedly compressing the patient's chest. These hands will give you a visual indication that CPR is in progress. When you stop CPR, the hands will disappear.

The patient is supine to best display the equipment that is in use. This position does not represent the position in which the patient is found nor does it necessarily represent the position in which you would place the patient to perform proper care. Questions about positioning of each of the patients will be found in the study guide lessons.

Above the patient visual, a display indicates whether you are "On Scene" or "In Transit."

## Running Log

The running log is seen on the right side of the interface (shown below).

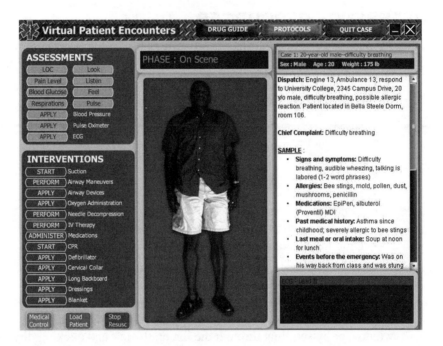

When you first enter the patient care interface after watching the video, the log will display the initial dispatch that you heard, as well as the patient's chief complaint and history in SAMPLE/OPQRST format. You should read this information before making any assessment or intervention decisions because doing so will provide a more total picture than the video alone.

Once you begin making assessments, the data and observations appear in the running log in the order that you perform the assessments below the **Now On Scene** heading. This running log lets you know what is happening with the patient and, by reassessing, what is changing about the patient.

All interventions that you perform are also recorded in the running log. Interventions are always listed in italics to distinguish them from assessments. All the choices you make within the steps of the intervention wizards are recorded on the log; for example, when administering medications, the dose and the route are recorded in addition to the drug name.

Certain messages appear in the log in red type, either to notify you that something drastic has changed about your patient or to let you know that something you tried to do was not possible and why. For example, if your patient becomes unconscious while you are treating him or her, you may receive the message, "Your patient's condition has changed. You need to reassess," or "Patient is exhibiting seizure activity." If you were to try to defibrillate while performing CPR, you would receive a message such as, "Unable to perform defibrillator unsync shock, you are still doing CPR." Once you stop CPR, you can defibrillate.

As your running log fills up with more and more information, you can use the scroll bar on the right to scroll up and down, perhaps to compare assessment data before and after a particular intervention.

Note that the case number and complaint, as well as the patient's gender, age, and weight, are listed for your information across the top of the running log.

Below the running log, an ECG display appears. As mentioned earlier, this display depicts Lead II of a 3-lead ECG.

# REFERENCE RESOURCES

Across the top of the interface, you will see a blue button marked **DRUG GUIDE** and a yellow button labeled **PROTOCOLS**, which can be used as reference resources.

Clicking **DRUG GUIDE** will open a new window in which you can review the following information about medications from the Emergency Drug Index in your textbook:

- Class
- Trade names
- Description
- Onset and duration
- Indications
- Contraindications
- Adverse reactions
- Drug interactions
- How supplied
- Dosage and administration
- Special considerations

You can look up a drug either by typing its generic name in the search field at the top of the window or by scrolling through the list on the left and clicking directly on its name. To close the drug guide window, click on the **X** in the upper right corner.

Clicking **PROTOCOLS** opens a different window that displays a menu of 23 protocols that were developed in accordance with your textbook and the 1998 National Standard Curriculum for the EMT-Paramedic. One or more of these protocols will be appropriate for each of the 15 cases found in this program. Simply click on the name of the protocol you want to open. Note that each protocol is divided into sections by scope of practice. Although the protocols will not tell you exactly what to do, keep in mind that they should put you on the right track if you have selected protocols that are relevant to the patient you are treating.

To return to the listing of protocols, click on **Return to List**. To close the protocols window, click on the **X** in the upper right corner.

# SUMMARY MENU

Three ways are provided to navigate to the summary menu, two of which you already know about; that is, by clicking **Unload Patient** while in transit or by clicking **Stop Resusc** after you have been given permission to do so by medical control. The third way is by clicking the red **QUIT CASE** button to the right of the **PROTOCOLS** button. Use this button to leave a case when you want to skip it or to switch to another case. Many study guide lessons may only require you to watch the video and read the history before answering the questions, in which case you will be directed to simply quit the case.

The summary menu itself offers four choices as described below:

**LOG**—Click the **Log** button to view, save, or print the log from the case you just completed. The information that was recorded in the running log during patient care is now displayed full screen for you to review easily (shown below).

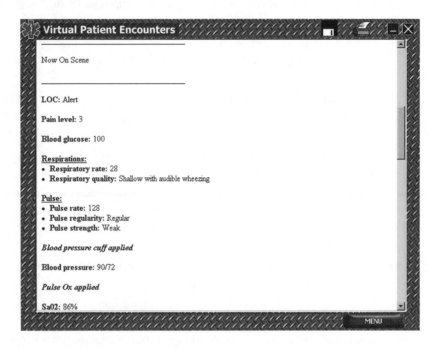

All of the summative lessons will instruct you to review the log of your patient care while answering questions in the study guide. Click the icon of the floppy disk in the upper right corner to save your log as a rich text file, or click the icon of a printer to print out a hard copy. Be prepared for your instructor to ask you to submit your logs for his or her evaluation. Click **MENU** in the lower right corner to return to the summary menu.

**RESTART**—Click the **Restart** button to return to the patient selection screen. Be aware that unless you printed or saved a copy of your log from the case you just completed, a record of what you did will not be available to retrieve.

**CREDITS**—Click the **Credits** button to display a listing of all the people and organizations that contributed to the development of the simulation software. Click **RETURN TO MENU** to return to the summary menu.

**EXIT**—Click the **Exit** button to close the entire Virtual Patient Encounters program. As with clicking **RESTART**, be aware that unless you printed or saved a copy of your log from the case you just completed, no record of what you did will be available to retrieve.

## TIPS FOR USING VIRTUAL PATIENT ENCOUNTERS

Last, the following tips will improve your experience with Virtual Patient Encounters and can enhance your knowledge and prepare you for facing the uncertainty of the streets.

1. Always read the assigned chapter(s) before attempting the study guide lessons.

2. Keep your textbook handy as a reference while you work through the lessons.

3. Take your time—things in the program are not happening in real time. Reflect on your next action before you perform it.

4. Be sure to think about the appropriate sequence of actions. In real life, many assessments and interventions will happen simultaneously. When working in this program, you have to perform things one step at a time. For example, if you elect to intubate, you will have to stop bag-mask ventilation first.

5. Do not assume that others are performing certain skills or assessments as they would on a real call. You must specifically identify each assessment and intervention to be performed on the call.

6. Use the running log to review and reflect on what you have done so you can choose your next intervention or assessment.

7. Watch for the key messages (in red type) that may appear in the running log to indicate that the patient's condition has changed drastically. Failure to see one of these messages can lead you down the wrong path.

8. Just as you would in real life, reassess often, particularly after any significant intervention.

9. Because you do not interact with a live patient, you will not have benefit of the information and clues that you would normally have. Things such as how the patient feels (except for pain scale), his or her body language, and additional environmental clues will not be available. Simply use the information that you have and make the best judgments you can, based on the information you are given.

10. When you use the software program, follow the bulleted directions provided in the lessons and answer the relevant questions.

11. In some cases, you may think that an intervention or drug dose is appropriate but not available. Make the best choice available. This will prepare you for the "real world" of EMS where everything you need is also not available. Sometimes you have to improvise and do the best you can with what you have. The ability to make the most with the least is often what makes a great paramedic.

12. As previously mentioned, the protocols follow the guidelines in your textbook—sometimes these will vary from your local protocols. Discuss any variations and the reasons for them with your instructor.

13. The exact nature of illness or injury may not be perfectly clear in all cases. In other cases, you may have a pretty clear clinical impression, but you might not have any interventions that can correct the patient's problem. This scenario also mirrors real EMS practice. Simply perform the best interventions at your disposal and transport the patient when appropriate. Limitations in the prehospital setting will always occur.

We hope that Virtual Patient Encounters will be just one more tool to build your knowledge and improve your critical thinking ability as you move toward your goal to becoming a paramedic. Best wishes and good luck!

# Optional Online Resources

Virtual Patient Encounters (VPE) is a unique learning tool for you and your students. In addition to your students' study guide with simulation software and this instructor's Implementation Manual, you also have the option of using this product online within **Elsevier's Evolve Learning System**.

The following VPE resources are available online:

- **Online Study Guide**—If you wish, you can have your students complete their study guide lessons online instead of using the printed study guide. You can choose one of two user modes:

    **Discussion Mode** allows you to view your students' answers to completed study guide exercises, along with the correct answers for each exercise. This mode also allows you to provide feedback to your students or to request that a student redo and resubmit the assignment.

    **Grade Mode** also allows you to view your students' answers to completed study guide exercises, along with the correct answers for each exercise; however, in this mode you can assign grades to students' work, which can then be sent to each student individually and also deposited into your online grade book.

- **Online Test Bank**—This feature lets you create quizzes and examinations to test students' knowledge and critical thinking abilities.

- An electronic version of this Implementation Manual is available.

## REQUESTING VPE RESOURCES ON EVOLVE

### Technical Requirements

To use the above resources online, you will need access to a computer that is connected to the Internet and equipped with web browser software that supports frames. For optimal performance, it is recommended that you have speakers and use a high-speed Internet connection. However, slower dial-up modems (56 K minimum) are acceptable.

Please follow these steps to request VPE Resources:

1. Go to the Evolve site (http://evolve.elsevier.com/Sanders/paramedic/instructor).
2. On the Evolve page, locate the VPE listing and click on **Register for these free resources**.
3. Follow the instructions provided by the step-by-step Registration Wizard.

All requests for resources on Evolve must be approved by the sales representative in the requestor's area. This is done to verify the identity of the person making the request. After submitting your request, please allow up to 2 business days for approval of domestic requests (in the United States). Please allow up to 7 business days for approval of all international requests. Requests being submitted during a weekend or holiday may take longer to be approved.

Once your request has been approved, you will receive an e-mail message containing your user name, password, login instructions, and course ID.

### Enrolling Your Students

The VPE Resources on Evolve are provided in a "course" that is specific to you and your students. Once your VPE Resources request has been approved and your course has been created, you will need to enroll your students into your specific course.

Please follow these steps:

1. Gather your students' first names, last names, and e-mail addresses. You will also need your user name, password, and course ID.
2. Go to the instructor home page on Evolve (located at http://evolve.elsevier.com/Sanders/paramedic/instructor).
3. Click on **Help & Support** located on the menu at the top of the screen. Then click on **Submit Class Roster**.
4. Follow the instructions provided by the step-by-step **Roster Wizard**.

Completing the **Submit Class Roster Wizard** will create a user name and password for each user submitted and enroll each user into your specific course. While completing the Wizard, you will have the option of e-mailing the user name and password to each student automatically or having a list sent to you only.

*Note:* You can use the Submit Class Roster Wizard to enroll as many users as necessary into your course-as many times as you need. You do not have to enroll all users at the same time. Additional instructors can be enrolled into your course through this same process.

Once your students are enrolled into your specific course, they will need to login at http://evolve.elsevier.com/login. Your course will be included in the list of courses in which they are enrolled. Their login information is provided in the e-mail message they receive if you chose to have their account information sent automatically to them. If you chose to have their account information sent to you only, you will need to provide each student with his or her user name and password.

## SUPPORT INFORMATION

**Live support** is available to customers in the United States and Canada from 7:30 AM to 7 PM (CST), Monday through Friday by calling 1-800-401-9962. You can also send an email to evolve-support@elsevier.com.

There is also **24/7 support information** available on the Evolve website (http://evolve.elsevier.com), including:

- Guided Tours
- Tutorials
- Frequently Asked Questions (FAQs)
- Online Copies of Course User Guides
- And much more!

# Emergency Medical Services Systems: Roles and Responsibilities

## Assignment

### Prerequisites:

- Complete Chapter 1, Emergency Medical Services Systems: Roles and Responsibilities, in *Mosby's Paramedic Textbook, Revised Third Edition.*
- Complete Chapter 1 in the workbook for *Mosby's Paramedic Textbook, Revised Third Edition.*
- Complete any skills or laboratory studies pertinent to this lesson.
- Read the "Getting Started" and "Orientation to Virtual Patient Encounters" sections in the *Virtual Patient Encounters Study Guide* (if this is the first lesson being attempted).

### Student assignment:

- Complete Lesson 1 in the *Virtual Patient Encounters Study Guide* after you have reviewed the topic in class.

## Topic Review

### Objectives:

*On completion of this lesson, the student will be able to perform the following:*

- Describe how the attributes of the professional paramedic are demonstrated during patient care activities.

### Review the following topics with your students before they complete the lesson:

- The paramedic provides emergency care based on advanced assessment skills and the formulation of a field impression.
- Training and performance standards help define emergency medical services (EMS) professionals.
- Professionalism refers to the way a person follows professional standards.
- Attributes of the professional paramedic include integrity, empathy, self-motivation, appearance and personal hygiene, self-confidence, communications, time management, teamwork and diplomacy, respect, patient advocacy, and careful delivery of service.
- Primary responsibilities of the paramedic include preparation, response, scene and patient assessment, recognition of injury or illness, patient management, appropriate patient disposition, transfer, and documentation and returning to service.

1

- Secondary responsibilities of the paramedic include community involvement, support of primary care efforts, advocate citizen involvement in EMS, leadership activities, and personal and professional development.
- Paramedics work under a medical director as part of a complex multidisciplinary team that relies on the fact that each paramedic will practice in a competent, professional manner.

## ■ Follow-Up

### *Assignment follow-up from the previous class:*

- What problems, if any, did you have with your assignment?
- What questions do you have?

### *In-class activities and discussion questions:*

- What effect might the professional behavior of the paramedics have on the outcome of this call?
- Describe some strategies to establish communication with a non–English-speaking patient.
- Why would continuing education benefit the paramedic on a call such as this one?
- How will you find out what the specialty resource hospitals are in your area?

### *Summary assessment:*

- Administer the quiz related to this lesson (Evolve resources, instructor's test bank).

## ■ STUDY GUIDE ANSWERS

### EXERCISE 1 ■ *Case 10: 25-year-old female—abdominal pain*

1. Describe specific behaviors you observed of the paramedics on this call that demonstrate the attributes of the professional paramedic. If the attribute is not seen on this call, then write *not observed.*

| Attribute | Specific Behavior Observed on this Call |
|---|---|
| Integrity | **Not observed** |
| Empathy | **When the neighbor stated the patient had lost two babies before, the paramedic stated, "I'm sorry to hear that."** |
| Self-motivation | **Not observed** |
| Appearance and personal hygiene | **Both paramedics appear fit, neat, clean, and very professional in hygiene grooming and uniform.** |
| Self-confidence | **Both paramedics seem to have predefined roles and confidently move to perform care.** |
| Communications | **The attending paramedic is patient and polite. He explains what they are going to do before doing it. Rather than pulling away the cloth over the patient's eyes, he asks her neighbor to have the patient remove it. Before he begins his examination, he asks the neighbor to "tell her we'll be touching her."** |

| Attribute | Specific Behavior Observed on this Call |
|---|---|
| Time management | **Not observed** |
| Teamwork and diplomacy | **He and his partner work together seamlessly without having to tell each other what to do. The attending paramedic also works well with the translator neighbor. He is patient and polite.** |
| Respect | **He shows respect by listening without interrupting and by telling the patient what he will be doing before he does it.** |
| Patient advocacy | **The video mentioned that the patient did not have any money. The paramedics did not change their evaluation or demeanor based on this information.** |
| Careful delivery of service | **Both paramedics do not appear to be rushing. They move confidently and carefully toward their patient-care goals.** |

2. On this case, why will it be important for the paramedic to have a good working knowledge of hospital designation and categorization?

   **This patient will need obstetrical services, if they are available in this region (high-risk obstetrical services, if they are available). The paramedic should recognize this need and know exactly how to get the patient to these services in a timely manner.**

3. Describe what type of online or off-line medical direction the paramedics may need on this call.
   a. Online medical direction:

      **The paramedics will contact the receiving facility to let them know that a high-risk patient is being transported. In addition, because this type of call is uncommon, the paramedic may consult with online medical direction regarding drug treatment in this case.**

   b. Off-line medical direction:

      **The paramedics may have protocols or standing orders that allow administration of the drugs that this patient needs without online contact.**

## EXERCISE 2 ■ *Case 9: 22-year-old female—assault*

4. Describe why each of these professional attributes is important on this call. Then, describe whether you observed them in the brief time you had to observe the paramedics on the call.

| Attribute | Specific Behavior Observed on this Call |
|---|---|
| Integrity | **An aspect of integrity that is essential on this type of call is accurate and thorough documentation. This factor will be important if criminal prosecution of the persons who assaulted her is sought. This was not observed.** |
| Empathy | **Empathetic behavior is important to the emotional well-being of a patient who has been assaulted. These paramedics were caring, respectful, and calm.** |
| Self-motivation | **On this type of call, the self-motivated paramedic would be thorough and observe for small details that may be critical to patient care or** |

| Attribute | Specific Behavior Observed on this Call |
|---|---|
| | procecution. He or she would ensure the patient is taken to a hospital with a sexual assault examination specialist (if available in the area) and call ahead to alert the hospital so the patient would not have a long wait. This is not observed on this call. |
| Appearance and personal hygiene | A neat professional appearance can inspire the patient's trust and confidence. Both paramedics are neat, clean, and look professional. |
| Self-confidence | A patient who has been assaulted is often fearful. The EMS crew must appear self-confident and sure of their actions to instill a sense of trust in the patient. These paramedics, though very low keyed, appear confident by their organized, calm, orderly approach to the patient. |
| Communications | Effective communication is essential on this call. The paramedics must listen to the reports of others (police, patients) carefully and interpret the information correctly. Their approach must convey calmness, empathy, and confidence to the patient who is fearful. They must then be able to relay the information clearly to the receiving facility. After the call, the paramedic must communicate the events of the call effectively in writing on the patient report. Then, if asked to testify, he or she must relate the findings on the call clearly and accurately. The paramedics on this call listened attentively to the report of the police and to the patient's comments. They did not interrupt or rush the comments of others. They asked appropriate questions of the patient without prying into areas potentially upsetting to the patient that would not affect EMS care. |
| Time management | Performing EMS tasks on the scene thoroughly while being mindful that definitive treatment for the patient is at the hospital is always important so as to minimize scene time. Not enough of this call was observed to determine the on-scene time. |
| Teamwork and diplomacy | A case such as this involves multijurisdictional resources to work together effectively for a positive patient outcome. The paramedics must focus on medical care while the police objective will be to provide safety, obtain facts related to prosecution, and to apprehend the perpetrators. The paramedics and police appeared to work together collaboratively on this case. |
| Respect | Some individuals have a tendency to judge the events of an alleged sexual assault and to display behaviors or make comments questioning the circumstances of the assault. These behaviors can be detrimental to the emotional recovery of the patient. These paramedics demonstrated respect by their body language and verbal communication with the patient. |
| Patient advocacy | In this case, patient advocacy is important as it relates to maintaining patient confidentiality and to treating the patient fairly with respect and consideration regardless of the paramedic's beliefs. The paramedics allowed the female officer to remain with the patient. |
| Careful delivery of service | In this case, careful delivery of service is important as it relates not only to both care of the patient's injuries and to relieving her pain, but also as it relates to preservation of evidence. The paramedics are beginning to methodically begin their examination in the brief video clip that is observed. |

# The Well-Being of the Paramedic

## ■ Assignment

### Prerequisites:

- Complete Chapter 2, The Well-Being of the Paramedic, in *Mosby's Paramedic Textbook, Revised Third Edition.*
- Complete Chapter 2 in the workbook for *Mosby's Paramedic Textbook, Revised Third Edition.*
- Complete any skills or laboratory studies pertinent to this chapter.
- Read the "Getting Started" and "Orientation to Virtual Patient Encounters" sections in the *Virtual Patient Encounters Study Guide* (if this is the first lesson being attempted).

### Student assignment:

- Complete Lesson 2 in the *Virtual Patient Encounters Study Guide* after you have reviewed the topic in class.

## ■ Topic Review

### Objectives:

*On completion of this lesson, the student will be able to perform the following:*
- Discuss measures that can be taken to reduce the incidence of paramedic injury or illness related to an emergency medical services (EMS) call.
- Identify wellness practices that minimize the risk of injury on the job.

### Review the following topics with your students before they complete the lesson:

- Physical and emotional well-being are both critical aspects of the paramedic's health that must be maintained to deliver care safely and effectively.
- Proper nutrition, which includes adequate intake of water, is a critical aspect of personal wellness.
- Physical fitness helps increase personal wellness and increases resistance to injury.
- Aspects of fitness the paramedic should maintain include cardiovascular endurance, muscle strength, and muscular flexibility.
- Proper use of body mechanics when lifting a heavy object or person is essential to prevent injuries while on the job.
- Get extra help if needed. Look where you are walking. Move forward, if possible, with short steps. Bend at the hips and knees. Use the legs to lift. Keep the load close to the body. Use a wide stance to distribute weight more evenly and to lower the center of gravity.

- Infectious disease prevention includes practicing good personal hygiene, getting proper immunizations, and following universal (standard) precautions.

# Follow-Up

### Assignment follow-up from previous class:

- What problems, if any, did you have with your assignment?
- What questions do you have?

### In-class activities and discussion questions:

- Have two students come to the front of the room, and then place an object on the ground and ask them to pick it up. After they do, ask the class to critique the students' use of proper body mechanics when they picked up the object. Review the components of body mechanics, and emphasize the need to use these strategies when lifting objects of any size so they become a habit.
- Have each student write on an index card an activity that he or she routinely uses to relieve stress. Have students pass the cards to the front of the room. Discuss some of the activities, and ask the students whether they believe that the activities promote good health and what benefits (or disadvantages) the activity may have.

### Summary assessment:

- Administer the quiz related to this lesson (Evolve resources, instructor's test bank).

# STUDY GUIDE ANSWERS

### EXERCISE 1 ■ Case 12: 57-year-old male—man down

1. What lifting techniques did you observe the paramedics demonstrate that should reduce the risk of back injury on the job?

   **When the paramedic lifts the cot, he or she bends and lifts with the legs and keeps the back straight. The partner assists by lifting the legs. The paramedic also holds the load close to the body.**

2. How can paramedics reduce their susceptibility to heat-related illness while on the job?

   **During high-heat periods, paramedics should wear the lightest weight uniform permitted and wear sunblock, sunglasses, and a hat if long periods of exposure to sun are anticipated. They should drink plenty of fluids before and after calls to maintain hydration, and they should be sure to eat nutritious meals at appropriate intervals.**

3. What measures were the paramedics using to reduce their risk of exposure to blood or bloody body fluids? Discuss the reasons you believe these measures are adequate or the reasons they are not.

   **The paramedics are wearing gloves and eye protection. This precaution appears to be adequate because no evidence can be found that a high risk of splash or spray of blood or bloody body fluids exists on this call.**

**EXERCISE 2** ■ *Case 1: 20-year-old male—difficulty breathing*

4.  List measures you can take to minimize the risk of injury to the crew or the patient if the patient is conscious but cannot walk down the stairs.

    **If the patient is conscious, then a stair chair can be used to bring him or her safely down the steps. The paramedics should secure the patient firmly in the chair and communicate often as they move the patient slowly down the stairs.**

5.  What individual characteristics about the paramedics did you note that might reduce the patient's risk of injury or illness?

    **Both paramedics look muscular and fit, as if they work out to maintain optimal physical conditioning. This regimen will prepare them to perform their job safely and can give a sense of well-being to help manage the psychologic stress associated with EMS.**

6.  If the paramedics worked several consecutive shifts and were severely sleep deprived, how could that condition influence their performance on this call?

    **Sleep deprivation can lead to impaired driving, with an increased risk of vehicle collision, inattention that can lead to a fall when lifting or carrying a patient, or faulty or slow decision-making ability in a life-threatening situation.**

7.  What measures, aside from gloves and other standard precautions, should the paramedics take to reduce their risk of getting or spreading infectious disease?

    a.  Measures to take while on the job:

    **On the job, the EMS crew should be sure to wash their hands thoroughly with soap and water each time gloves are removed and at the end of each call. Equipment in the ambulance should be properly cleaned or disinfected after each patient, depending on the nature of the call. Dispose of sharps immediately after use, never use a one-handed recap technique, use safety needle devices when available, and properly dispose of soiled equipment.**

    b.  Preventive measures to take that protect them on every call:

    **Off-the-job activities include maintaining good personal health by eating a nutritious diet, exercising, and getting plenty of sleep. In addition, the paramedic should get appropriate immunizations to reduce the risk of acquiring a communicable disease (hepatitis B, tetanus, diphtheria, influenza). A tuberculin skin test should be performed every year (or more often in high-risk regions) to detect exposure to tuberculosis early.**

# Injury Prevention

## ■ Assignment

### Prerequisites:

- Complete Chapter 3, Injury Prevention, in *Mosby's Paramedic Textbook, Revised Third Edition*.
- Complete Chapter 3 in the workbook for *Mosby's Paramedic Textbook, Revised Third Edition*.
- Complete any skills or laboratory studies pertinent to this chapter.
- Read the "Getting Started" and "Orientation to Virtual Patient Encounters" sections in the *Virtual Patient Encounters Study Guide* (if this is the first lesson being attempted).

### Student assignment:

- Complete Lesson 3 in the *Virtual Patient Encounters Study Guide* after you have reviewed the topic in class.

## ■ Topic Review

### Objectives:

*On completion of this lesson, the student will be able to perform the following:*
- Apply Haddon's matrix to selected cases to identify factors that contribute to injury.
- Relate injury prevention principles to selected cases.
- Identify resources available to develop an injury-prevention program.

### Review the following topics with your students before they complete the lesson:

- Emergency medical services (EMS) providers play an important role in injury prevention activities.
- Three factors influence injury and disease: host, agent, and environment. In injury, these factors are referred to as the injury triangle.
- Haddon's matrix divides these three factors into a timeline that identifies factors that play a role at each phase. These time frames are pre-event, event, and postevent phases.
- Three strategies are used to prevent injuries, referred to as the 3 *E*s: education, enforcement, and engineering. Because injury-prevention measures in engineering are passive, it is the most effective.
- EMS providers play an essential role in injury prevention. They are often seen as experts and advocates for the patient. In addition, EMS providers are trusted and welcomed into homes, schools, and community organizations.

- The role of EMS in injury prevention should begin with protection from job-related injury. Other roles include promoting data collection, using injury data, obtaining support for injury prevention activities, and conducting injury-prevention activities.

- On-scene education can be effective because patients are motivated to learn. This is called the teachable moment. It involves three steps: (1) observe the scene, (2) gather information, and (3) make an assessment. Methods used include discussion, demonstration, and documentation.

- Prevention programs begin by gathering information to determine the scope and costs associated with an injury-prevention program. Many community resources can provide valuable information to identify the need for injury prevention and to help plan the program. These resources include trauma registry data, local public safety agencies, your own department database, federal agencies, and other resources.

- Community health education can be provided verbally using written or static methods or using dynamic methods. Regardless of the method, the delivery method must use appropriate language and communication methods that are relevant to the intended audience.

# Follow-Up

### Assignment follow-up from previous class:

- What problems, if any, did you have with your assignment?
- What questions do you have?

### In-class activities and discussion questions:

- Give some examples of calls during which a teachable moment may occur. How would you convey this education?
- What type of injury or illness prevention methods have been most effective to assist you (the student) in making good, safe choices?
- How can you determine if the intended audience will understand your health and safety education printed materials?

### Summary assessment:

- Administer the quiz related to this lesson (Evolve resources, instructor's test bank).

# ▪ STUDY GUIDE ANSWERS

### EXERCISE 1 ▪ *Case 7: 8-year-old male—submersion*

1. Complete the following table to relate the components of Haddon's matrix to this call.

| Phase | Host | Agent | Environment |
|---|---|---|---|
| Pre-event | Children may not have good judgment relative to their abilities to control depth of the dive. This child was playing with friends and was inattentive as to the risks of shallow diving. | The pool markings may not indicate the depth of the water. If a diving board existed, then it might have been broken, causing the injury. Surfaces around the edge of the pool may be unsafe. | The bottom of the pool might be hard concrete. A large crowd of friends may be present (easy to miss someone who is submerged). Water for submersion may exist. |

2. Discuss how the three *E*s of injury prevention could be applied to prevent children from drowning.

   a. Education:

   Children should be taught about the dangers of diving into unfamiliar or shallow water, about swimming without adult supervision, and about the benefit of formal swim lessons.

   b. Enforcement:

   Pool owners might be required to have lifeguards present to prevent injuries by enforcing pool rules and intervening if a problem should occur.

   c. Engineering:

   Measures include high fencing with a gate that can be opened only by an adult, locked pool area unless supervision is present, and an audible pool alarm that will alert adults if a child falls into the water.

3. If the child in this case survives his injury, predict the costs (not actual dollars) that will be associated with this injury.

   Associated costs include ambulance transport, emergency department and hospital care, intensive care unit charges, spinal cord and head injury rehabilitation, medical equipment such as wheelchairs and assistive devices, home modifications to permit transfers, specialized vehicles to permit transport, follow-up medical care, cost of complications associated with long-term care of spinal injury, and potential wages lost resulting from limitations related to spinal cord and head injury.

**EXERCISE 2 ■ *Case 2: 56-year-old female—fell***

4. What pre-event factors contribute to fall-related injuries in older adults?

| Host | Agent | Environment |
|------|-------|-------------|
| Medications, visual impairment, decreased balance, medical illness | Improper home or vehicle maintenance, household items placed on high shelf where climbing is needed | Poor lighting in the home, loose carpet |

5. What resources would you use to find out the incidence and cost of older adult fall-related injuries in your community?

   **Local EMS agency, local trauma registry can provide information related to elderly falls, local medical direction. The Centers for Disease Control and Prevention collects injury data.**

6. How will you determine how many older adults live in your community?

   **Census data and local library**

7. Where can you ask for money to help fund your program?

   **Your employer, local trauma center, community service organizations, and public and private grants**

8. You decide to develop a written flyer as part of your injury-prevention program. How can you make sure that it will be effective and understood by your intended audience?

   **Be sure to write the information in a format that is understandable (write at the appropriate grade level and language) and engaging to your intended audience. Before you publish the material, have several people from your intended audience read the flyer and give feedback about readability and how well it conveyed your intended message.**

9. How can you measure the effectiveness of your program?

   **You can track data after the interventions and compare them to the data before the interventions to see if a measurable decrease in injuries has occurred after you implemented your program.**

# Medical/Legal Issues

## ■ Assignment

### Prerequisites:

- Complete Chapter 4, Medical/Legal Issues, in *Mosby's Paramedic Textbook, Revised Third Edition.*
- Complete Chapter 4 in the workbook for *Mosby's Paramedic Textbook, Revised Third Edition.*
- Complete any skills or laboratory studies pertinent to this chapter.
- Read the "Getting Started" and "Orientation to Virtual Patient Encounters" sections in the *Virtual Patient Encounters Study Guide* (if this is the first lesson being attempted).

### Student assignment:

- Complete Lesson 4 in the *Virtual Patient Encounters Study Guide* after you have reviewed the topic in class.

## ■ Topic Review

### Objectives:

*On completion of this lesson, the student will be able to perform the following:*

- Relate the legal principles of assault, battery, and false imprisonment to the restraint issue in Case 8.
- Discuss how consent is obtained when caring for the patient in Case 8.
- Apply the elements of negligence to a variation of this case.

### Review the following topics with your students before they complete the lesson:

- Competent patients have a right to choose to accept or deny care. By agreeing to the care after understanding it, they give informed consent. When they tell the EMS provider that they consent or when they provide their consent in writing, it is expressed consent.
- In some circumstances, care is provided without expressed consent. This includes cases involving mentally incompetent adults and prisoners or arrestees. EMS providers should be familiar with local laws and protocols with regard to both patient groups.
- If a patient is transported using physical force without his or her consent, the EMS provider may be accused of assault, battery, and false imprisonment.
- False imprisonment occurs when a person is detained without just cause. This could occur if an EMS provider transports a competent adult without consent against his or her will.
- Making threats to restrain a competent patient physically could be construed as assault.

- Physical contact with a person without consent or any legal cause is battery.
- Before an EMS provider restrains a patient, provides unwanted care to a patient, or transports a patient without consent and against the patient's wishes, he or she should ensure that this is within legal boundaries. This protects both the paramedic and the patient.
- Negligence is the failure to act as a reasonable, prudent paramedic would act in similar circumstances.
- Four components of negligence must be proven: (1) a duty to act existed; (2) a breach of duty occurred; (3) injury (damage) occurred; and (4) the breach was the proximate cause of the damage.

## ■ Follow-Up

### Assignment follow-up from previous class:

- What problems, if any, did you have with your assignment?
- What questions do you have?

### In-class activities and discussion questions:

- What is the punishment for conviction of assault, battery, or false imprisonment in your area?
- How can you decrease your risk of being accused of assault, battery, or false imprisonment?
- Have the class discuss some examples of negligent behaviors that might occur on an EMS call.

### Summary assessment:

- Administer the quiz related to this lesson (Evolve resources, instructor's test bank).

## ■ STUDY GUIDE ANSWERS

### EXERCISE 1 ■ Case 8: 38-year-old male—suicide attempt

1. What observations from the patient's initial assessment made it acceptable to restrain and transport him against his will?

   **This patient was not competent and was a danger to himself, he threatened suicide, and he was displaying incoherent speech with delusional thoughts and flight of ideas.**

2. Research the involuntary admission laws in your state. How long can this patient be held against his will? Who has the authority to hold him for longer than the initial phase?

   **Involuntary admission for psychiatric evaluation varies by state. It may be 72 hours or shorter or longer, depending on the situation. In many instances, a judge must order holding a patient for a longer period.**

3. What type of consent applies in this case?

   **You should refer to local protocols to determine what type of consent would apply here. Because he needs emergency care related to a suicide threat, and because his behavior leads you to believe that he is incompetent, he is treated much as you would a minor.**

4. Should you ask the patient about his wishes regarding care and transportation?

   **Asking the patient is always advisable.**

5.  You fail to assess the restrained patient and he vomits, aspirates, and dies. List the four elements needed to prove negligence, and explain how your actions would satisfy each of these four elements.

| Element | Why it Is Satisfied or Not Satisfied |
| --- | --- |
| Duty to act | You assumed care of the patient and had a duty to act. |
| Breach of duty | If proof exists that you failed to perform your duty or performed it in an inappropriate manner, then a breach has occurred. For example, if you did not monitor a restrained patient adequately, then you may have breached your duty. |
| Damage | The patient died. |
| Proximate cause | If proof can be found that your failure to monitor the patient adequately resulted in his death, then proximate cause may be established. |

6.  In the previous example, did the negligence result from malfeasance, misfeasance, or nonfeasance? Explain your answer.

    **When you do not perform a required act or duty, the situation is termed nonfeasance, which, in this example, is the cause of negligence.**

# Ethics

## ■ Assignment

### Prerequisites:

- Complete Chapter 5, Ethics, in *Mosby's Paramedic Textbook, Revised Third Edition.*
- Complete Chapter 5 in the workbook for *Mosby's Paramedic Textbook, Revised Third Edition.*
- Complete any skills or laboratory studies pertinent to this chapter.
- Read the "Getting Started" and "Orientation to Virtual Patient Encounters" sections in the *Virtual Patient Encounters Study Guide* (if this is the first lesson being attempted).

### Student assignment:

- Complete Lesson 5 in the *Virtual Patient Encounters Study Guide* after you have reviewed the topic in class.

## ■ Topic Review

### Objectives:

*On completion of this lesson, the student will be able to perform the following:*

- Describe strategies to resolve ethical conflicts.

### Review the following topics with your students before they complete the lesson:

- Ethics is the field that relates to right and wrong, duty and obligation, principles and values, and character.
- Paramedics must often make difficult ethical choices. These decisions may sometimes conflict with personal values.
- Ethical problem analysis can include asking yourself if you have ever encountered this situation before; if you have time, deliberating with co-workers or medical direction about the issue; and considering a test for the ethical dilemma.
- The impartiality test asks if you would accept the decision if you were in the patient's place.
- The universalizability test asks if you would be comfortable with this action in other similar situations.
- The interpersonal justifiability test asks if you can defend and justify your actions to others.

- Answer the following four questions when resolving ethical dilemmas:
  1. What is in the patient's best interest?
  2. What are the patient's rights?
  3. Does the patient understand the situation?
  4. What is the paramedic's professional, legal, and moral accountability?
- Common ethical issues in emergency medical services (EMS) include those relating to allocation of resources, decisions surrounding resuscitation, confidentiality, and consent.

# Follow-Up

### Assignment follow-up from previous class:

- What problems, if any, did you have with your assignment?
- What questions do you have?

### In-class activities and discussion questions:

- Would factors such as this patient's obesity influence your decision regarding resuscitation?
- How will your decision to transport or your choice of hospital destination be influenced by a patient's ability to pay or by her immigrant status? Consider what you would do if the patient asks you, "Do I really need to be transported? I don't have any money. I can't afford any more bills."

### Summary assessment:

- Administer the quiz related to this lesson (Evolve resources, instructor's test bank).

# STUDY GUIDE ANSWERS

### EXERCISE 1 ■ Case 2: 56-year-old female—fell

1. As you interview the patient, her husband comes in and says, "Oh, I forgot to tell you, she has a *Do Not Resuscitate* order. She does not want anything to be done if she stops breathing. It's right here in the living room. I'll go and get it." The patient nods *yes*.

   a. He goes to get the *Do Not Resuscitate* order, and she stops breathing. What should you do?

   **Laws regarding Do Not Resuscitate (DNR) vary from state to state. You should follow the laws from your state. Generally, you should have a written DNR order that is consistent with your state and district policies if you elect to execute the DNR order. Online medical direction can also be consulted regarding the appropriate action to take in these cases. In most instances, the law requires that you resuscitate if no written order is present.**

   b. He returns and says he is having trouble finding the order. What action should you take?

   **Generally, if no documentation can be found, then resuscitation would continue. If you have sufficient team members, then have someone explain your obligation to follow state law and comfort him.**

c. What ethical principles apply to this situation?

**You wish to help the patient or at least do no harm. If you cannot confirm her wishes, then you should err on the side of treating her. You also have an ethical responsibility to avoid interfering if a patient has an incurable illness. However, you have little history from either the patient or husband in this case to make this determination.**

### EXERCISE 2 ■ *Case 14: 65-year-old male—difficulty breathing*

2. You assess this patient and determine that he is in severe distress and that he may be having a heart attack. When you tell your partner to get the stretcher so that you can transport the patient, the patient refuses to go, saying, "I won't leave my dog. There's no one else to take care of him." Despite your best efforts to persuade the patient to go to the hospital, he refuses transport.

a. What ethical principles apply to this situation?

**The ethical principle in this situation would revolve around consent. Ethically and legally, patients have a right to consent or withhold consent for medical treatment and, in the case of EMS, transport.**

b. What strategies can you use to resolve this dilemma?

**You should make every effort to resolve this situation in a manner that is ethical, legal, and benefits the patient. Determine if you can make acceptable alternative arrangements for the dog. Explain to the patient the seriousness of his condition. You can consult with medical direction to determine if they can offer advice.**

### EXERCISE 3 ■ *Case 10: 25-year-old female—abdominal pain*

3. If you discover that this patient is an undocumented alien with no health insurance, how will it influence your treatment or transport decisions?

**A patient's ability to pay or his or her legal status should have no bearing on treatment or transport decisions.**

4. If the patient tells you that she has no money and does not wish to be transported, what actions should you take?

**You must explain to the patient the medical reasons she needs transport, as well as the risks to both the patient and her unborn child if she declines transport. You must also verify through the translator that the patient understands the risks of refusal if she continues to decline transport. If possible, online contact with a Spanish-speaking physician from medical direction should be made to speak directly with the patient. Money should not influence your decisions related to her care and transport.**

# Review of Human Systems

## ■ Assignment

### Prerequisites:

- Complete Chapter 6, Review of Human Systems, in *Mosby's Paramedic Textbook, Revised Third Edition*.
- Complete Chapter 6 in the workbook for *Mosby's Paramedic Textbook, Revised Third Edition*.
- Complete any skills or laboratory studies pertinent to this chapter.
- Read the "Getting Started" and "Orientation to Virtual Patient Encounters" sections in the *Virtual Patient Encounters Study Guide* (if this is the first lesson being attempted).

### Student assignment:

- Complete Lesson 6 in the *Virtual Patient Encounters Study Guide* after you have reviewed the topic in class.

## ■ Topic Review

### Objectives:

*On completion of this lesson, the student will be able to perform the following:*

- Use directional terms appropriately to describe wound locations.
- Relate the observed injuries to the anatomic structures involved.
- Describe alterations in the physiologic condition that should be anticipated based on the wounds observed.

### Review the following topics with your students before they complete the lesson:

- For emergency medical services (EMS) providers to communicate clearly, they must use accepted medical directional terms appropriately and consistently, which is important for the appropriate on-going care of the patient and for medical-legal reasons.
- Directional terms are always used as they relate to a patient who is in the anatomic position: standing erect, feet and palms facing the examiner.
- Knowledge of the anatomic feature that lies under the surface of the skin is important when trying to predict blunt or penetrating injuries. Additionally, paramedics must be able to predict how normal physiologic features of these structures will be altered by the injuries.

- Important structures in the head and neck include the brain and spinal cord, major blood vessels, the upper and part of the lower airway structures, sense organs, and some endocrine glands (pituitary, thyroid).
- The thorax also contains many structures that are vital for survival. Injuries to the chest are likely to involve the lungs or heart. Additionally, the esophagus, spine, and many large blood vessels lie in this region.
- Many vascular structures lie in the abdomen. The liver and spleen are both highly vascular and, if injured, can lead to life-threatening shock. The kidneys are in the retroperitoneal space, and many organs of the digestive and endocrine system are in the abdomen as well. The pancreas, stomach, intestines, and adrenal glands are located here.
- The major great vessels (aorta and vena cava) pass through the abdomen and can cause rapid death if injured.

## ■ Follow-Up

### Assignment follow-up from previous class:

- What problems, if any, did you have with your assignment?
- What questions do you have?

### In-class activities and discussion questions:

- Explain how the proper use of medical terminology would be essential if this case were to go to court.
- What is the importance of predicting which anatomic structures are positioned under the surface of penetrating wounds?

### Summary assessment:

- Administer the quiz related to this lesson (Evolve resources, instructor's test bank).

## ■ STUDY GUIDE ANSWERS

### EXERCISE 1 ■ Case 11: 32-year-old male—gunshot wounds

1. Describe the location of the injuries using proper anatomic terminology.
   a. The neck wound was located **lateral** to the midline of the neck.
   b. The chest wound was located **superior** to the nipple and **inferior** to the clavicle.
   c. The abdominal wound was located **superior** and **lateral** to the umbilicus. The abdominal wound was located in the **right upper** quadrant of the abdomen.
   d. The patient was found in the **supine** position.
2. Predict which anatomic structures should be located under each wound:
   a. Neck wound:

   **Arteries or veins of the neck (carotid artery or jugular veins), airway structures (trachea), spine or spinal column**

b. Chest wound:

**Lung, blood vessels in the chest (intercostals, subclavian, or others), possibly the spine. If the path of the bullet went medially, then the great vessels of the chest might be involved.**

c. Abdominal wound:

**Liver, small bowel, mesentery, diaphragm, if the bullet traveled medially the inferior vena cava. If it penetrates inferior and posterior, then the kidneys might be involved.**

3. Predict alterations in the normal physiologic condition of body systems that may be affected by these wounds:

a. Neck wound:

**If the blood vessels are involved, then hemorrhagic shock may result. If the airway is penetrated, then the patient may have impaired ventilation caused by blood in the airway or an alteration in the mechanics of breathing. If the spinal cord is involved, then the patient may have quadriplegia and spinal cord shock.**

b. Chest wound:

**If the lung is involved, then the patient may have pneumothorax, hemothorax, or tension pneumothorax. If the blood vessels of the chest are involved, then hemorrhagic shock may result.**

c. Abdominal wound:

**Hemorrhagic shock may result from liver or blood vessel damage. Renal failure can occur if the kidney is involved. Peritonitis may result from perforation of the bowel.**

4. Using the dermatome map on p. 117 of your textbook, predict the location where the patient would lose sensation if the neck wound penetrated the spinal cord.

**If cord injury at C7 was complete, then the patient may have sensation in his pinky and ring finger but not the rest of his hand. He will have some sensation in the posterior medial aspect of his arm but none in the rest of his arm. He will not have sensation below the clavicle.**

# General Principles of Pathophysiology

## ■ Assignment

### Prerequisites:

- Complete Chapter 7, General Principles of Pathophysiology, in *Mosby's Paramedic Textbook, Revised Third Edition*.
- Complete Chapter 7 in the workbook for *Mosby's Paramedic Textbook, Revised Third Edition*.
- Complete any skills or laboratory studies pertinent to this lesson.
- Read the "Getting Started" and "Orientation to Virtual Patient Encounters" sections in the *Virtual Patient Encounters Study Guide* (if this is the first lesson being attempted).

### Student assignment:

- Complete Lesson 7 in the *Virtual Patient Encounters Study Guide* after you have reviewed the topic in class.

## ■ Topic Review

### Objectives:

*On completion of this lesson, the student will be able to perform the following:*

- Predict alterations in pH that will be present based on the initial case information.
- Predict physiologic responses that will occur as the body compensates for acute blood volume loss.

### Review the following topics with your students before they complete the lesson:

- The body produces respiratory and metabolic acids during normal metabolism. The body must maintain acid and base balance within a very narrow range to achieve normal functions. Normal pH of the blood is 7.35 to 7.45.
- Excess acidity can result when carbon dioxide ($CO_2$) is not excreted normally through the respiratory system. This situation can occur from any disease or injury that impairs normal ventilation and causes the $CO_2$ level to rise. The normal range of $CO_2$ is between 35 and 45.
- To treat respiratory acidosis, the paramedic must take rapid action to open the airway and improve ventilation.
- When ventilation is impaired, oxygenation is often also decreased. Normal partial pressure of oxygen ($PO_2$) ranges from 80 to 100 mm Hg. Impaired ventilation, decreased ambient inhaled $O_2$ levels, or respiratory diseases that interfere with diffusion of oxygen into the alveoli can cause decreased $PO_2$.

**21**

- To treat decreases in oxygenation, the paramedic should ensure a patent airway and adequate ventilation and supply supplemental $O_2$. Additionally, any underlying injury or illness that inhibits diffusion of oxygen across the respiratory membrane should be addressed.
- When blood volume drops, the body's baroreceptors and chemoreceptors sense the change, and immediately trigger a series of compensatory mechanisms aimed at restoring normal perfusion.
- These mechanisms include sympathetic responses, the central nervous system ischemic response, the adrenal medullary mechanism, renin-angiotensin-aldosterone mechanism, vasopressin mechanism, reapsorption of tissue fluids, and the discharge of blood from the venous sinuses of the spleen.
- Activation of these mechanisms increases circulating blood volume, increases peripheral vascular resistance, increases heart rate and stroke volume, and dilates bronchioles. Each response is aimed at improving oxygenation to the tissues. They produce the signs and symptoms of shock that the paramedic will observe before any drop in blood pressure is detected.

# ■ Follow-Up

### *Assignment follow-up from previous class:*

- What problems, if any, did you have with your assignment?
- What questions do you have?

### *In-class activities and discussion questions:*

- Describe the compensatory mechanisms the body uses when it senses a sudden drop in blood volume as seen in gastrointestinal bleeding or after penetrating chest trauma.
- Describe the importance of having a fundamental knowledge of acid-base balance when you are delivering bag-mask ventilation to a patient.
- What effect does cardiac arrest have on the body's acid-base balance?

### *Summary assessment:*

- Administer the quiz related to this lesson (Evolve resources, instructor's test bank).

# ■ STUDY GUIDE ANSWERS

### EXERCISE 1 ■ *Case 1: 20-year-old male—difficulty breathing*
### *Case 13: 5-month-old male—unresponsive*

1. What alterations in blood gasses would you expect to find in each of these cases based on the initial information you are given for these calls?

| Case | Partial Pressure of Oxygen (PO$_2$) | | Partial Pressure of Carbon Dioxide (PCO$_2$) | | pH | |
|---|---|---|---|---|---|---|
| | Alteration | Based On | Alteration | Based On | Alteration | Based On |
| 1 | Decreased PO$_2$ | Impaired ventilation; cyanosis | Increased PCO$_2$ | Impaired ventilation; air trapping caused by bronchospasm | Decreased pH | Lactic acidosis from hypoxia and increased CO$_2$ |
| 13 | Decreased PO$_2$ | Apnea | Increased PCO$_2$ | No ventilation or circulation | Decreased pH | Lactic acidosis related to hypoxia and hypoperfusion |

2. What actions will you need to take to correct these alterations?

   a. Case 1:

   **Open the airway by administering medicines to dilate the bronchioles and decrease inflammation (epinephrine, methylprednisolone, albuterol), administer high-concentration oxygen.**

   b. Case 13:

   **Open the airway; assist ventilations with high-concentration oxygen; begin cardiopulmonary resuscitation; perform treatment aimed at restoring circulation.**

### EXERCISE 2 ■ *Case 5: 40-year-old male—vomiting blood*

3. Assume that, after assessing this patient, you determine he that has the following vital signs: blood pressure (BP) 100/84, pulse (P) 128, respiration (R) 28, skin is pale and cool. Is this compensated or uncompensated shock? Explain your answer.

   **Compensated shock. Tachycardia, tachypnea, and skin pallor are present, but the BP is still within normal limits.**

4. Describe how the compensatory mechanisms activated in response to the patient's acute blood loss produce some of the physical findings of your examination.

| Compensatory Mechanism | Action | Physical Finding |
|---|---|---|
| Increased sympathetic stimulation | Epinephrine and norepinephrine are released and stimulate alpha and beta receptors | Pale skin, increased heart rate |

| Compensatory Mechanism | Action | Physical Finding |
|---|---|---|
| Adrenal medullary mechanism | Releases epinephrine and norepinephrine; stimulates alpha and beta receptors | Pale, cool skin; increased heart rate |
| Renin-angiotensin-aldosterone mechanism | Angiotensin II increases peripheral vascular resistance. | Pale, cool skin |
| Vasopressin mechanism | Vasopressin (antidiuretic hormone) causes peripheral vasoconstriction. | Pale, cool skin |

5. Which compensatory mechanisms increase intravascular volume during shock?

**The aldosterone produced by the renin-angiotensin-aldosterone mechanism causes the kidneys to retain water. The vasopressin (antidiuretic hormone) mechanism enhances reabsorption of water in the kidneys. Low capillary hydrostatic pressure promotes reabsorption of interstitial fluid into the blood vessels. Blood stored in the venous sinuses of the spleen is released in the circulating blood volume in shock.**

# Life Span Development

## ■ Assignment

### Prerequisites:

- Complete Chapter 8, Life Span Development, in *Mosby's Paramedic Textbook, Revised Third Edition*.
- Complete Chapter 8 in the workbook for *Mosby's Paramedic Textbook, Revised Third Edition*.
- Complete any skills or laboratory studies pertinent to this lesson.
- Read the "Getting Started" and "Orientation to Virtual Patient Encounters" sections in the *Virtual Patient Encounters Study Guide* (if this is the first lesson being attempted).

### Student assignment:

- Complete Lesson 8 in the *Virtual Patient Encounters Study Guide* after you have reviewed the topic in class.

## ■ Topic Review

### Objectives:

*On completion of this lesson, the student will be able to perform the following:*
- Determine if the children in these scenarios fall within normal age-specific developmental guidelines.
- Discuss the effect of emotional development on wellness.
- Distinguish between illness and injuries that occur within specific age ranges.

### Review the following topics with your students before they complete the lesson:

- Newborns weigh 3 to 3.5 kg at birth. You should expect their weight to double within 4 to 6 months and triple by 1 year.
- Infants' airways are short and narrow. They will breath faster if exposed to infection or stress and, as a result, can lose body heat and fluids.
- Their nervous systems develop quickly. Initially they depend on reflexes. By age 2 months, they can recognize faces; by age 10 months, they can recognize their own names.
- Motor development during the first year progresses from initially being unable to hold up his or her own head to sitting upright in a chair at 6 months, sitting without assistance by 8 months, pulling up to standing at 9 months, and walking at 1 year.
- The immune system is enhanced by passive immunity during the first 6 months after birth. Maternal antibodies protect infants from some diseases.

- Infants recognize their primary caregivers and may smile at that person within 2 or 3 months. By 9 months, they may have separation anxiety when separated from their caregivers.
- When evaluating an infant, the paramedic should determine if the history is reasonable based on the infant's predicted developmental stage. Some injuries and illnesses should not appear in this age group.

# ■ Follow-Up

### *Assignment follow-up from previous class:*

- What problems, if any, did you have with your assignment?
- What questions do you have?

### *In-class activities and discussion questions:*

- Show a brief scene from a movie (e.g., Cheaper by the Dozen) or television series (e.g., Seventh Heaven), and ask the class to identify age-specific differences in physical and emotional development of the characters.
- For the cases presented in this chapter, ask the class what differences they would have seen had the patient been 5 years older or 5 years younger.

### *Summary assessment:*

- Administer the quiz related to this lesson (Evolve resources, instructor's test bank).

# ■ STUDY GUIDE ANSWERS

### EXERCISE 1 ■ *Case 13: 5-month-old male—unresponsive*

1. Does this infant's weight (16 lb) seem appropriate for a baby of his age? Explain your answer.

   **Normal birth weight is approximately 7 pounds. At 1 year, the child would be approximately 3 times birth weight. At 5 months, 16 pounds would be within the expected range.**

2. Would you have expected a 5-month-old infant to sleep through the night, or is the mother's story questionable?

   **By approximately 5 months, children sleep through the night without food; therefore her story would be believable.**

3. If you resuscitate this baby, then what vital signs would you expect as normal for his age?

   **You would expect the following vital signs for a 5-month-old child: pulse approximately 120 bpm, respirations approximately 30 per minute.**

4. If you resuscitate this baby and he were to become fully conscious, how would you expect him to respond to his mother?

   **You should expect that he would recognize his mother and reach out to her.**

5. How is a baby this age protected against disease?

   **The baby has some passive immunity up to approximately 6 months of age.**

6. If you resuscitate this child, stroke the outside of his foot, and his toes fan up toward his head, how would you interpret these finding? What assessment have you performed?

   **This finding would be normal for a child this age. The toes would not point down until the child is walking. This action assesses the Babinski reflex.**

7. Which of the following illnesses or injuries would you expect to find in a 5-month-old infant? If you said you would not expect it, then explain your answer.

| Illness or Injury | Expected in a 5-Month-Old Infant | If You Said No, Explain Why |
|---|---|---|
| Father says infant burned his feet stepping into the tub. | **No** | **A child of this age would be unable to pull to standing or climb into a tub.** |
| Pertussis | **No** | **He should still have passive immunity.** |
| Fell while walking and hit his head. | **No** | **Walking would be unusual for a child of this age.** |
| Choked on a bead. | **Yes** | **Children this age can move objects to their mouths.** |

## EXERCISE 2 ■ *Case 6: 16-year-old female—unknown medical*

8. Do this patient's vital signs fall within the expected normal range for her age? Explain your answer.

   **No. Blood pressure should be 100 to 120 mm Hg systolic; her blood pressure is 78/56 mm Hg. Heart rate for her age should be 55 to 105 bpm; her heart rate is 134 bpm. Respiratory rate should be 12 to 20 breaths/min; her respiratory rate is 10 and shallow.**

9. What sexual characteristics should have developed in a girl of this age? Explain why this patient may have delayed development in this area.

   **She should have well-developed breasts, have reached menarche, and have developed hair in her pubic area and under her arms. However, patients with anorexia may have delayed sexual development related to low body weight.**

10. What emotional developmental characteristics would predispose a girl of this age to develop anorexia?

    **Teenagers are often very concerned about their body image. A large number of teenagers are obsessed with body weight. This circumstance can lead to eating disorders such as anorexia and severe depression.**

11. What factors may lead you to believe that this situation is a suicide attempt?

    **Depression and suicide ideation is common in patients of this age. You found a partly filled bottle of antidepressant pills next to the patient. This call has a high probability of being a suicide attempt.**

# Therapeutic Communication

## ■ Assignment

### Prerequisites:

- Complete Chapter 9, Therapeutic Communication, in *Mosby's Paramedic Textbook, Revised Third Edition*.
- Complete Chapter 9 in the workbook for *Mosby's Paramedic Textbook, Revised Third Edition*.
- Complete any skills or laboratory studies pertinent to this chapter.
- Read the "Getting Started" and "Orientation to Virtual Patient Encounters" sections in the *Virtual Patient Encounters Study Guide* (if this is the first lesson being attempted).

### Student assignment:

- Complete Lesson 9 in the *Virtual Patient Encounters Study Guide* after you have reviewed the topic in class.

## ■ Topic Review

### Objectives:

*On completion of this lesson, the student will be able to perform the following:*

- Identify therapeutic communication techniques used by the paramedics in selected cases.
- Recognize barriers to effective communication, and identify strategies that may be used to overcome them.

### Review the following topics with your students before they complete the lesson:

- Therapeutic communication is one of the most important skills a paramedic can master. Good therapeutic communication can facilitate an accurate history, diffuse anger and emotional situations, and help ensure customer satisfaction.
- Communication has six elements: the source, encoding, the message, decoding, the receiver, and feedback. If a problem exists with any of the elements, then the intended message may not be transmitted.
- Verbal communication can be improved by using fewer words, speaking simply, avoiding the use of vague phrases, using examples to illustrate a point, repeating key points, avoiding the use of technical jargon, speaking at a normal speed, and avoiding long pauses.
- Internal factors that promote effective communications include liking others, empathy, and an ability to listen actively.

- Effective listening techniques include facing patients while they speak, maintaining natural eye contact, assuming an attentive posture, and leaning forward.
- The paramedic should try to control external factors to foster an environment in which therapeutic communication can occur. Strategies include ensuring privacy and minimizing interruptions, maintaining eye contact, and presenting yourself in a professional manner.
- To maximize your chance of an effective interview, ask open-ended questions in a narrative form, encourage the patient to talk, and do not limit the responses.
- Establishing a good rapport with the patient is important. Try to put him or her at ease, and let him or her know you are trying to ensure the patient's best interests. Recognize verbal and non-verbal cues that indicate the patient needs help. Show compassion. Ensure that the patient understands what is happening by speaking at his or her level. Show confidence so the patient trusts your ability to perform your job.

# ■ Follow-Up

### Assignment follow-up from previous class:

- What problems, if any, did you have with your assignment?
- What questions do you have?

### In-class activities and discussion questions:

- Give the group a piece of paper with a series of statements. Ask students to read it using a variety of body language (arms crossed versus arms open) and a variety of verbal inflections (voice quiet and slow versus voice loud and fast). Ask students how the patient might perceive the message in each situation. (Example statement: "Why did you call us today?")

### Summary assessment:

- Administer the quiz related to this lesson (Evolve resources, instructor's test bank).

## ■ STUDY GUIDE ANSWERS

### EXERCISE 1 ■ *Case 2: 56-year-old female—fell*

1. Review the steps for effective communication involved in the ladder of listening. Describe whether you observed each step in this case.

|   | Techniques for Effective Listening | How the Techniques Are Demonstrated |
|---|---|---|
| L | Look at the patient. | The first rescuer makes good eye contact with the patient's husband and the second rescuer with the patient. |
| A | Ask more questions to clarify answers. | Both paramedics asked more questions in a nonthreatening manner. |
| D | Do not interrupt. | Both paramedics listened attentively for answers without interrupting. |
| D | Do not change the subject. | Neither paramedic changed the subject. |
| E | Empathize with the speaker. | No verbal demonstration of empathy took place, although the paramedics listened actively. |
| R | Respond to what is said verbally and nonverbally. | Paramedics nodded their head to acknowledge information was received. |

2. What barrier to effective therapeutic communication existed in this case?

   **The patient was critically ill and too dyspneic to respond completely. Her husband had very limited information to give the paramedics.**

3. How can paramedics adapt to this barrier most effectively?

   **Ask closed-ended questions. Minimize the number of questions to only those that are essential. Ask the patient to nod *yes* or *no* rather than speaking because she is struggling to breathe.**

### EXERCISE 2 ■ *Case 9: 22-year-old female—assault*

4. Describe the paramedic's communication with this patient as it relates to the following:
   a. Listening:

   **The paramedics get to the patient's eye level, keep a comfortable distance from the patient, and listen attentively.**

   b. Patience:

   **Her jaw injury is causing her to speak slowly. The crew never rushes her; rather, the crew waits to ensure that she completes her answers.**

   c. Providing privacy:

      **They interview the patient in a room with just the police officer. In this case, allowing the police officer to remain with the patient is likely prudent, given that she has allegedly been sexually assaulted and may be uncomfortable if left alone with two male attendants. The police officer stated that she had developed a rapport with the patient; therefore, in this case, this circumstance represents an effective use of resources.**

   d. Eye contact:

      **The paramedics kneel down to her level and are attentive, maintaining eye contact throughout the interview.**

   e. Personal dress:

      **Both paramedics appear professional, with crisp, clean uniforms.**

   f. Touch:

      **No touch is evident during the initial interview. Because this patient was assaulted, activities that involve touching the patient should be performed cautiously and only after explaining to the patient what is to be done.**

5. What barriers to effective therapeutic communication existed on this call?

   **The patient had injuries to her jaw and face that made speech painful and slow. In addition, her emotional state may have impaired normal communication. Her assailants allegedly gave her drugs. Depending on the nature, strength, and duration of the drugs, they might impair her ability to communicate normally.**

6. What strategies can paramedics use to overcome these barriers?

   **The paramedics can allow the female officer to remain with the patient. Ask closed-ended questions that require *yes* or *no* answers to minimize her pain. Administer pain medicine cautiously to make her more comfortable (the patient may have been given some drugs by her assailants). This approach should make speech less painful.**

7. If the police officer had not been present, how might the officer's absence affected the interview?

   **Had the female officer not been present, the patient may have been fearful and less likely to provide information. In the absence of a female, the male paramedics might establish rapport with careful therapeutic communication—a female may not always be present.**

## EXERCISE 3 ■ *Case 10: 25-year-old female—abdominal pain*

8. What barrier to communication was present on this case?

   **The patient did not appear to speak any English.**

9.  Explain the techniques in Box 9-7 on page 223 of *Mosby's Paramedic Textbook* that the paramedic used with the interpreter to obtain appropriate information.

    **The paramedics introduced themselves through the interpreter, spoke to the interpreter but then looked at the patient as the interpreter was questioning her and as she responded to the interpreter, asked questions that needed only one response at a time as opposed to complex questions, did not interrupt the patient or interpreter, did not discuss the patient's condition in front of the interpreter without explaining the comments to the patient, and used simple language when asking the questions.**

10. If the interpreter had not been present, could the interpreter's absence have changed your clinical impression? Explain your answer.

    **Had the interpreter not been present, the crew would not have known the patient's signs and symptoms, due date, pregnancy history, nature of her pain, prenatal care, or other medical history. They may have simply thought that she was in labor rather than pre-eclamptic and at risk for abruption.**

11. What techniques could have been used to obtain information in the absence of an interpreter?

    **Had the interpreter not been present, another neighbor or source for interpretation should be sought. Translation aids such as pocket guides can be used. Some hospitals have translation services that are available over the telephone. Your emergency medical services system or dispatch center may have a translation policy for situations such as this one.**

# History Taking

## ■ Assignment

### Prerequisites:

- Complete Chapter 10, History Taking, in *Mosby's Paramedic Textbook, Revised Third Edition*.
- Complete Chapter 10 in the workbook for *Mosby's Paramedic Textbook, Revised Third Edition*.
- Complete any skills or laboratory studies pertinent to this lesson.
- Read the "Getting Started" and "Orientation to Virtual Patient Encounters" sections in the *Virtual Patient Encounters Study Guide* (if this is the first lesson being attempted).

### Student assignment:

- Complete Lesson 10 in the *Virtual Patient Encounters Study Guide* after you have reviewed the topic in class.

## ■ Topic Review

### Objectives:

*On completion of this lesson, the student will be able to perform the following:*
- Evaluate a patient within the context of additional information about the patient's history.
- Value the importance of patient history as part of the assessment process.

### Review the following topics with your students before they complete the lesson:

- History taking often provides information essential to establish a field impression.
- The components of the patient history include the chief complaint, history of present illness, significant medical history, and current health status.
- The chief complaint is the reason for a 9-1-1 call. The complaint can be verbal or nonverbal. Chief complaints often involve pain, abnormal function, a change in the patient's normal state, or an unusual observation.
- History of present illness includes information related to the onset and origin of the problem, factors that provoke or palliate the complaint, the quality of pain, the location of the pain or problem and whether it radiates to another area, the severity of the pain, and the time symptoms have persisted.
- Significant medical history can play an important role in the current situation. Medical history should include general health status, significant medical illnesses, surgeries, psychiatric illnesses, social problems, and hospitalizations.

- Current health status can focus on medications and allergies, as well as changes in the daily activities such as the patient's last menstrual cycle, last bowel movement, and last oral intake.
- In an emergency setting, obtaining an accurate and complete patient history often presents challenges. These challenges can include patients who are silent, overly talkative, afflicted by multiple symptoms, angry, intoxicated, or developmentally delayed.

# ■ Follow-Up

### *Assignment follow-up from previous class:*

- What problems, if any, did you have with your assignment?
- What questions do you have?

### *In-class activities and discussion questions:*

- Why is effective history taking a critical element of prehospital assessment?
- What are some possible consequences of ineffective history taking?
- Why might history-taking techniques vary from call to call?

### *Summary assessment:*

- Administer the quiz related to this lesson (Evolve resources, instructor's test bank).

# ■ STUDY GUIDE ANSWERS

### EXERCISE 1 ■ *Case 6: 16-year-old female—unknown medical*

1. What physical findings would you anticipate if, after examining the pill bottle or talking with the patient's parents, you discover the following information? What clinical impression or impressions would this information give you?

| Information | Impressions | Physical Findings |
| --- | --- | --- |
| She has been using oxycodone (OxyContin) and was released from drug rehabilitation last week. | Narcotic overdose | Pupil constriction, depressed level of consciousness and ventilation |
| Her parents just discovered that she is bulimic. Her weight is 60 pounds. Her physician called when he received her laboratory results and told her parents to call an ambulance; he would arrange for a direct admission to the intensive care unit (ICU). | Electrolyte imbalance, dehydration related to bulimia, or both | Dry mucous membranes, tenting of the skin, dullness of the eyes, decreased level of consciousness, pale skin, hypotension, tachycardia. If electrolyte imbalance is present, then dysrhythmias or CNS problems may occur. |
| She wrote a suicide note; the bottle was filled with digoxin yesterday. | Overdose of cardiac glycoside | Severe arrhythmias leading to cardiac arrest; bradycardia, heart block leading to asystole |

| Information | Impression | Physical Findings |
|---|---|---|
| Her parents tell you she is diabetic and has been vomiting for 2 days. | **Diabetic ketoacidosis** | **Dull eyes, dry mucous membranes, acetone odor on breath, skin tenting, tachycardia, hypotension. Arrhythmias from severe acidosis may occur if untreated.** |

### EXERCISE 2 ■ *Case 14: 65-year-old male—difficulty breathing*

2. What form of questioning did the paramedic use to begin the interview of the patient?

   **Open-ended questioning.**

3. After discovering that the patient was having difficulty communicating, how did the paramedic change his questioning?

   **Direct questioning.**

4. What nonverbal communication techniques did you notice during the initial assessment?

   **The paramedic knelt at the patient's level, looked directly at the patient, and kept his hand on the patient's arm after he assessed his pulse.**

5. What physical findings would you anticipate if you discover the following information? What clinical impression or impressions would you consider as significant?

| Information | Impressions | Physical Findings |
|---|---|---|
| He is drowsy, vomiting, dyspneic, and has a headache. His furnace has not been working correctly. | **Possible carbon monoxide toxicity** | **Tachycardia, oxygen saturation may be normal or decreased, decreasing mentation, elevated environmental carbon monoxide on gas meter. You should immediately take this patient out of the house to evaluate.** |
| He has noticed a cough with green sputum for several days. He is now febrile. | **Possible pneumonia** | **Discolored sputum, fever, diminished breath sounds, rhonchi or wheezes in localized area of lung; may develop sepsis and signs of shock.** |
| He has a history of severe emphysema and has developed sudden dyspnea with a sharp pain in the right side of his chest. | **Possible spontaneous pneumothorax related to emphysematous bleb rupture** | **Decreased oxygen saturation, diminished breath sounds on one side. If tension pneumothorax develops, then signs of shock, jugular venous distention, and tracheal deviation may occur.** |

| Information | Impressions | Physical Findings |
|---|---|---|
| His home medicines include an Atrovent inhaler, Singulair, a Maxair inhaler, and prednisone that he says his physician prescribed 2 days earlier. | **Exacerbation of chronic obstructive pulmonary disease or asthma** | **Tachycardia, tachypnea, wheezes, diminished breath sounds, pulsus paradoxus, accessory muscle use, decreased oxygen saturation, end-tidal carbon dioxide waveform with a shark fin appearance** |

# Techniques of Physical Examination

## ◼ Assignment

### *Prerequisites:*

- Complete Chapter 11, Techniques of Physical Examination, in *Mosby's Paramedic Textbook, Revised Third Edition.*
- Complete Chapter 11 in the workbook for *Mosby's Paramedic Textbook, Revised Third Edition.*
- Complete any skills or laboratory studies pertinent to this lesson.
- Read the "Getting Started" and "Orientation to Virtual Patient Encounters" sections in the *Virtual Patient Encounters Study Guide* (if this is the first lesson being attempted).

### *Student assignment:*

- Complete Lesson 11 in the *Virtual Patient Encounters Study Guide* after you have reviewed the topic in class.

## ◼ Topic Review

### *Objectives:*

*On completion of this lesson, the student will be able to perform the following:*

- Demonstrate physical examination techniques in the given scenario.
- Demonstrate the components of a comprehensive physical examination in the given scenario.
- Describe the general approach to a physical examination.
- Distinguish between normal and abnormal findings in a mental status assessment.
- Demonstrate physical examination techniques used for specific body regions.

### *Review the following topics with your students before they complete the lesson:*

- Four examination techniques that are commonly used in physical assessment include (1) inspection, (2) palpation, (3) percussion, and (4) auscultation.
- Inspection involves a visual assessment of (1) the overall appearance of the patient and environment and (2) each specific body region.
- The hands and fingers are used to perform palpation. Information such as temperature and the presence of masses, fluids, and crepitus are gathered using this examination technique. The presence of pain during palpation should also be carefully noted.

- Percussion, although not widely used, is a process during which the paramedic taps one finger against another to generate sounds from the underlying tissues. The noise produced will vary according to the type of underlying tissue and whether the structures under the percussed area are filled with air or fluid or whether the structure is a solid organ.

- Auscultation usually involves the use of a stethoscope to amplify body sounds. This technique is used to evaluate air movement in the lungs, blood flow through the heart valves, and bowel sounds. Auscultation takes practice to discriminate subtle sounds.

- Examination equipment should be appropriate for the size and type of patient. Equipment that is available for various sized patients includes blood pressure cuffs and some stethoscopes (e.g., fetoscopes).

- The mental status examination is one of the earliest evaluations performed and can provide valuable information regarding the patient's condition.

- Evaluation of the thorax should include inspection of all surfaces for injuries, as well as evaluate normal chest expansion and the use of accessory muscles during respiration. The chest is palpated to detect painful areas or the presence of asymmetry or detects. The chest is percussed from side to side and observed for variation from the normal resonance that should be heard over normal lungs. Breath sounds should be systematically auscultated for presence and quality, as well as to detect adventitious sounds that signal injury or disease.

- When evaluating the abdomen, it is first inspected and then auscultated before palpation or percussion. If the patient complains of abdominal pain, then the painful region is palpated last, using care to prevent unnecessary discomfort.

## ■ Follow-Up

### Assignment follow-up from previous class:

- What problems, if any, did you have with your assignment?
- What questions do you have?

### In-class activities and discussion questions:

- What are some consequences of incorrectly performing the physical examination?
- Why must you recognize normal findings for the physical examination in each body area?
- How will you perfect your skills of physical examination?

### Summary assessment:

- Administer the quiz related to this lesson (Evolve resources, instructor's test bank).

## ■ STUDY GUIDE ANSWERS

### EXERCISE 1 ■ PREPARATION ACTIVITY

1. Before you begin the simulation, recall the techniques of physical examination you will need to use. List and describe them below:
   a. **Inspection, carefully viewing or looking at all anatomic regions**
   b. **Palpation, using the sense of touch to feel for abnormalities**
   c. **Percussion, a technique used to evaluate the presence of air or fluid in body tissue**
   d. **Auscultation, using a stethoscope to assess body sounds produced by movement of various fluids or gases in organs or tissues**

## EXERCISE 2 ■ *Case 1: 20-year-old male—difficulty breathing*

2. What signs or symptoms should you anticipate with this type of complaint?

**Skin redness, swelling, itching, and hives; swelling around the eyes or mouth; airway narrowing with stridor; hypotension and other signs of shock; gastrointestinal upset with vomiting; bronchospasm leading to respiratory failure if untreated**

3. Describe a thorough assessment of James' chest.

**The patient's clothing should be removed to expose the chest. The chest wall should be inspected for symmetry on the anterior and posterior surfaces. The chest wall should then be palpated for pulsations, tenderness, bulges, depressions, crepitus, subcutaneous emphysema, unusual movement, and position. Percussion should be performed on the chest, listening closely for hyperresonance, dullness, or flat sounds. Using the diaphragm of the stethoscope, auscultation is best performed with the patient in an upright position.**

4. Why would you focus your physical assessment more on James' respiratory effort and thorax than on the rest of his body?

**James has a respiratory chief complaint; thus the assessment should be focused on the respiratory system and thorax.**

5. Describe your technique to auscultate James' thorax.

**Ask the patient to breathe in and out slowly through the mouth. Then, using the diaphragm side of a stethoscope, the posterior thorax should be auscultated in 10 places, first one side and then the next so as to compare lungs sounds. Both left and right midaxillary lines should be auscultated, comparing from left to right, moving from superior to inferior. Then the anterior surface of the chest should be auscultated, from the clavicles to the sixth intercostal space, comparing the left lateral with the right lateral sounds and moving superior to inferior.**

6. What sounds would you expect to hear as you auscultate James' thorax?

**Wheezing**

## EXERCISE 3 ■ *Case 2: 56-year-old female—fell*

7. What signs of distress do you see in this patient?

**Signs of cardiorespiratory insufficiency such as labored breathing, signs of pain such as sweating, anxiety, restlessness, and an anxious expression**

8. How would you describe her initial mental status examination?

**She is awake and alert but slow to respond. Whether she is oriented is difficult to determine from the initial video. Her severe dyspnea makes a thorough mental status examination difficult.**

9. What are your immediate assessment priorities for this patient?

**Rapid survey including rapid assessment of breathing status and vital signs. The patient should be moved (or the furniture moved, if possible) to permit better assessment and access to the patient.**

10. Which techniques of physical examination may need to be modified, based on your initial impression of this patient?

    **An *obese* or thigh-sized blood pressure cuff (i.e., sphygmomanometer) will need to be used. Heart sounds will often be muffled or diminished in the obese patient. Palpation of the apical pulse is difficult in obese patients.**

11. Based on your assessment of the patient, what type of illness or complaint do you suspect?

    **A cardiac complaint, possibly congestive heart failure**

### EXERCISE 4 ■ *Case 10: 25-year-old female—abdominal pain*

12. Describe the order in which you will perform examination techniques on the abdomen.

    **Inspection, auscultation, percussion, and palpation. The assessment should be done in this manner to avoid stimulating bowel sounds. If the abdominal pain is localized to one area, then this area should be palpated last.**

13. How will Connie's pregnancy affect your assessment of her abdomen?

    **The abdominal organs have shifted as the fetus grows. The size of the uterus increases from 70 to 1000 g and occupies the entire pelvic cavity. Connie's stomach will be displaced upward and laterally. Connie's liver is displaced posteriorly, upward and lateral to the right. Normal landmarks of the abdomen will be obscured by the growing fetus.**

# Patient Assessment

## ■ Assignment

### *Prerequisites:*

- Complete Chapter 12, Patient Assessment, in *Mosby's Paramedic Textbook, Revised Third Edition*.
- Complete Chapter 12 in the workbook for *Mosby's Paramedic Textbook, Revised Third Edition*.
- Complete any skills or laboratory studies pertinent to this chapter.
- Read the "Getting Started" and "Orientation to Virtual Patient Encounters" sections in the *Virtual Patient Encounters Study Guide* (if this is the first lesson being attempted).

### *Student assignment:*

- Complete Lesson 12 in the *Virtual Patient Encounters Study Guide* after you have reviewed the topic in class.

## ■ Topic Review

### *Objectives:*

*On completion of this lesson, the student will be able to perform the following:*

- Recall the components of patient assessment.
- Identify the essential patient assessment information from the scenario.
- Determine appropriate additional assessment needed.
- Discuss how to apply the phases of the patient assessment to each patient situation.

### *Review the following topics with your students before they complete the lesson:*

- The priorities of patient assessment include scene safety, recognition and management of life-threatening conditions, and identification of patients who need rapid stabilization and transport.
- Scene size-up and assessment are the first steps taken at any scene. This process includes determining the nature of the incident and the number of patients, assessing for hazards, initiating multiple-casualty incident set-up and triage if needed, requesting other resources if needed, identifying access and staging areas, and securing the scene.
- Appropriate personal protective equipment (PPE) should be selected based on the nature of the incident and the perceived or actual risks identified. This process always includes appropriate body substance isolation or universal precautions to prevent exposure to infectious diseases.
- Assessment priorities include initial assessment, focused history and physical examination, detailed physical examination, and ongoing assessment.

- Initial assessment includes forming a general impression of the patient, assessing and intervening for life-threatening conditions (by evaluation of level of consciousness, airway, breathing, and circulation), and identifying priority patients.
- Focused history and physical examination in a conscious medical patient will begin with a history and relevant physical examination. If the patient is unconscious, then a rapid head-to-toe examination should be performed.
- Rapid trauma physical examination is performed while spinal immobilization is maintained, which includes mental status assessment, a rapid head-to-toe examination, vital signs assessment, and patient history taking.
- Detailed physical examination would be performed to assess a specific injury or body area related to illness when no life threats are present or after the life threats have been managed.
- Ongoing assessment is performed at least every 5 minutes in critical or potentially unstable patients and every 15 minutes for others. This process includes reassessment of mental status, as well as airway, breathing, and circulation status, to reestablish patient priorities.

## ■ Follow-Up

### Assignment follow-up from previous class:

- What problems, if any, did you have with your assignment?
- What questions do you have?

### In-class activities and discussion questions:

- Why is the general impression a key element of the initial assessment?
- What are the main goals of the initial assessment?
- Explain the appropriate setting to perform a detailed patient assessment.

### Summary assessment:

- Administer the quiz related to this lesson (Evolve resources, instructor's test bank).

## ■ STUDY GUIDE ANSWERS

### EXERCISE 1 ■ PREPARATION ACTIVITY

1. List the assessment priorities and information needed in the initial assessment.

   **This includes general impression; level of consciousness; and airway, breathing, and circulation status.**

2. List the assessment priorities and information needed in the focused assessment.

   **This includes the chief complaint, history of present illness, medical history, and current health status. If the patient is unconscious, then perform a complete head-to-toe examination and assess vital signs.**

3. List the assessment priorities and information needed in the detailed assessment.

   **This includes a mental status general survey, head-to-toe examination, and baseline vital signs assessment.**

## EXERCISE 2 ■ *Case 1: 20-year-old male—difficulty breathing*

4. Why was it important to listen to the information provided by the emergency medical services responders and by the resident advisor for the dormitory?

    **Answers will vary. Without that information, the paramedics would not have known that epinephrine was already given.**

5. Using only the information you have from the initial dispatch and video information, identify the following:

    a. Your general impression of this patient:

    **He is a 20-year-old black male who appears to be in severe respiratory distress.**

    b. Patient's level of consciousness:

    **He is conscious and alert.**

    c. Patient's airway status:

    **His airway is patent.**

    d. Patient's oxygenation and respiratory status:

    **He has severe dyspnea, with wheezes that are audible without a stethoscope.**

    e. Patient's circulatory status:

    **He has a rapid heart rate and low blood pressure.**

6. Predict the life threats (if any) you will need to treat during the initial assessment of this patient. Explain your rationale.

    **His severe respiratory distress will need to be treated immediately. Circulatory life threats may be evident when the initial assessment is performed.**

7. List at least three possible causes of the symptoms presented in this case.

    **Symptoms may be related to an allergic reaction based on the present history. Other possible causes for dyspnea in a person of his age and with his history might be asthma or spontaneous pneumothorax.**

## EXERCISE 3 ■ *Case 2: 56-year-old female—fell*

8. What is your general impression of this patient?

    **This patient is a 56-year-old white female who is in severe respiratory distress.**

9. What difficulties did the team encounter in obtaining the initial patient information?

    **The patient's husband was a poor historian; he knew little about the patient's condition. When asked about her medications, her husband simply handed the crew a container of medicine. The patient was in severe respiratory distress and appeared to have altered consciousness such that she was unable to provide much information about her condition that was helpful to the emergency medical services (EMS) crew.**

10. How can the team overcome some of these difficulties?

**The EMS team can review the medications the husband gave them to determine what history the patient might have. The crew member interviewing the patient can ask closed-ended questions that require *yes* or *no* answers to minimize the energy the patient must expend to answer questions.**

11. What additional assessment information will be needed for this patient?

**The following assessments should be performed: breath sounds, vital signs, electrocardiogram (ECG) (12-lead ECG, if available), oxygen saturation, end-tidal carbon dioxide, blood glucose, and a quick head-to-toe examination to assess for signs of trauma related to her fall.**

12. List at least three possible causes of the signs and symptoms you have gathered up to this point for this case.

**Her signs and symptoms may be related to congestive heart failure, heart attack, exacerbation of chronic obstructive pulmonary disease, pulmonary embolus, or arrhythmia.**

### EXERCISE 4 ■ *Case 3: 7-year-old female—seizure*

13. Describe the components of the scene size-up that you assessed on this case.

| Component | Assessment |
| --- | --- |
| Nature | **Seizures** |
| Number of patients | **One** |
| Hazards identified | **Father is verbally aggressive and potentially violent; possible contagious infectious agent present** |
| Additional resources needed | **Police and possibly additional manpower to assist with care** |
| Are access or staging areas identified? | **No staging area is needed; access for stretcher and equipment will be difficult because of narrow space** |
| Is the area secure? | **Yes; however, potential exists to become hazardous (father)** |

14. During the video, the emergency medical services (EMS) team has gathered important assessment information. What is your general impression of this patient?

**The patient is a 7-year-old white female with seizure activity.**

15. Do you have enough information to determine if this case is related to illness or trauma? Explain your answer.

**At this point, the case appears to be a situation-related illness because of the history of fever, presence of rash, and previous illness. However, a more detailed assessment would be needed before traumatic head injury is ruled out as a cause of her seizure.**

**EXERCISE 5 ■** *Case 4: 64-year-old male—unknown medical*

16. What information did the EMS team obtain during the scene size-up?

| Component | Assessment |
| --- | --- |
| Nature | **Slurred speech, weak, disoriented** |
| Number of patients | **One** |
| Hazards identified | **None identified** |
| Additional resources needed | **Not unless his condition deteriorates** |
| Are access or staging areas identified? | **Patient is on upper level; no difficulty finding** |
| Is the area secure? | **Appears to be secure at this time; no apparent hazards** |

17. What additional assessment information should you obtain on this patient?

**Additional assessments needed include level of consciousness, airway, breathing, circulation, vital signs, focused physical examination including ECG (12-lead ECG, if available), oxygen saturation, and blood glucose analysis.**

18. Based on the history log and your observations from the video, list at least four current differential diagnoses for this case.

**Diabetic emergency, overdose, stroke, intoxication, unknown illness, or electrolyte abnormality**

**EXERCISE 6 ■** *Case 5: 40-year-old male—vomiting blood*

19. Describe your scene size-up and assessment for this call.

| Component | Assessment |
| --- | --- |
| Nature | **Male patient, vomiting blood, no apparent trauma** |
| Number of patients | **One** |
| Hazards identified | **Copious amounts of blood** |
| Additional resources needed | **Possible need for air medical transport (more information needed)** |
| Are access or staging areas identified? | **Apparent landing zone behind scene** |
| Is the area secure? | **Appears secure (no threats identified and law enforcement on scene)** |

20. What personal protective equipment (PPE) is appropriate for this type of call?

    **Face protection (goggles and face mask or face shield) is needed if persistent vomiting is present, gloves, and gown (to protect uniform).**

21. What life threats do you anticipate you will find in your initial assessment of this patient, based on the information from the scene size-up?

    **Patient appears unconscious with a large amount of blood around him. You should anticipate airway problems related to decreased consciousness and vomiting with possible blood and emesis in airway, breathing problems should be anticipated if he has vomited and aspirated, and circulation problems may be related to large blood loss.**

22. Based on the information you have, will this person be a priority patient? Explain your answer.

    **Unless an unusual explanation for this situation can be found, this person will be a priority patient because of the altered consciousness and gastrointestinal bleeding.**

23. What type of focused assessment will you perform on this patient?

    **Because the patient is unconscious, a rapid head-to-toe assessment should be performed.**

24. What type of detailed physical examination would be performed on this patient?

    **A detailed assessment will not likely be performed on this patient because he has immediate life threats that need to be addressed.**

25. What are the components of the ongoing assessment?

    **Ongoing assessment will include frequent (at least every 5 minutes) assessment of level of consciousness, airway, breathing, circulation, and vital signs.**

26. How often will you perform an ongoing assessment on this patient?

    **Ongoing assessment will performed at least every 5 minutes.**

### EXERCISE 7 ■ *Case 6: 16-year-old female—unknown medical*

27. What interventions should you anticipate having to perform during the initial assessment, based on the information you presently have?

    **You should anticipate having to perform airway maneuvers because she is apparently unconscious, to administer oxygen, and possibly to provide circulatory interventions (based on further assessment).**

28. What additional information will you need to determine whether this is a priority patient?

    **If you determine that she is unconscious and has a depressed gag or cough reflex, then she will be classified as a priority patient.**

29. List life threats that you would have anticipated if, instead of Elavil, the empty pill bottle had contained the following drugs:

| Drug | Life Threats Anticipated |
| --- | --- |
| Heroin | **Decreased level of consciousness, depressed respiratory drive and ventilation (possibly apnea), possible hypotension** |
| Digoxin | **Possible life-threatening dysrhythmias** |
| Xanax | **Decreased level of consciousness, worse if alcohol or other depressant taken concurrently** |
| Metoprolol | **Shock related to profoundly slow heart rate and hypotension** |
| Verapamil | **Shock related to vasodilation** |

### EXERCISE 8 ■ *Case 9: 22-year-old female—assault*

30. Did you note or do you expect to find any life threats related to level of consciousness, airway and breathing, and circulation?

**No life threat is immediately apparent. However, an airway problem might develop related to the trauma to her jaw or to the burns on her face. Possible shock might also be identified during the circulatory assessment related to the alleged substance that was injected by her assailants.**

31. What additional focused assessments should be performed on this patient?

**A focused assessment related to her injuries should be carefully performed. If further assessment determines the presence of a life threat, then a rapid head-to-toe examination would be performed.**

32. What factors will interfere with your ability to perform a complete assessment of this patient?

**The fact that this patient was assaulted and raped will cause you to be cautious in your evaluation. You must proceed with care and examine only specific areas needed to rule out life threats and to relieve her pain. Avoid examining areas that make the patient uncomfortable or fearful.**

### EXERCISE 9 ■ *Case 12: 57-year-old male—man down*

33. What sources of information relative to the situation and the patient's condition did you have on this call?

**The dispatcher, grounds crew, patient's friend, and patient**

34. What additional assessments should you perform on this patient?

**Additional assessments needed include level of consciousness, airway, breathing, circulation, vital signs, ECG, blood glucose, and oxygen saturation. The need for a focused examination will depend on initial findings.**

35. What preliminary information do you have about his airway, breathing, and respiration status?

    **He is apparently awake and breathing.**

36. Explain whether capillary refill would or would not be a reliable assessment to perform on this patient.

    **Capillary refill is generally not a reliable assessment in an older adult.**

37. List at least four possible causes of the signs and symptoms presented in this case.

    **Some differential diagnosis with this preliminary information might be intoxication, hypoglycemia, stroke, dysrhythmias, acute coronary syndrome, and heat-related illness.**

# Clinical Decision Making

## ■ Assignment

### Prerequisites:

- Complete Chapter 13, Clinical Decision Making, in *Mosby's Paramedic Textbook, Revised Third Edition*.
- Complete Chapter 13 in the workbook for *Mosby's Paramedic Textbook, Revised Third Edition*.
- Complete any skills or laboratory studies pertinent to this chapter.
- Read the "Getting Started" and "Orientation to Virtual Patient Encounters" sections in the *Virtual Patient Encounters Study Guide* (if this is the first lesson being attempted).

### Student assignment:

- Complete Lesson 13 in the *Virtual Patient Encounters Study Guide* after you have reviewed the topic in class.

## ■ Topic Review

### Objectives:

*On completion of this lesson, the student will be able to perform the following:*

- Apply clinical decision-making tools to selected virtual patient encounters (VPEs).
- Outline the elements of clinical decision making in emergency medical services (EMS) systems.

### Review the following topics with your students before they complete the lesson:

- Paramedics work in an unpredictable environment where they must gather and synthesize information quickly. Using this information, their judgment, and decision-making skills paramedics rapidly establish a field diagnosis from which their treatment plan follows.
- Concept formation is the first step in the decision-making process. It involves scene assessment, chief complaint, patient history and affect, initial assessment and diagnostic tests.
- Data interpretation follows concept formation. Relevant data must be gathered and interpreted within the proper context so decisions can be made.
- Application of principle flows from the decisions made in the data interpretation and concept formation phases. The paramedic selects the treatment plan based on the judgments made in those phases.
- Continual evaluation during (reflection in action) and after the intervention phase is essential so appropriate revisions to care can be made, if needed.

- After the event, reflection on action is provided by way of a run critique. Reflection provides an opportunity to evaluate the situation carefully and identify whether changes in approach would be warranted in future similar situations.
- The mental checklist for thinking under pressure includes stop and think, scan the situation, decide and act, maintain control, and continually reevaluate the patient.
- Six Rs are involved in putting the elements of decision making together on the call. They are Read the patient, Read the scene, React, Reevaluate, Revise the management plan, and Review performance.

## ■ Follow-Up

### *Assignment follow-up from previous class:*

- What problems, if any, did you have with your assignment?
- What questions do you have?

### *In-class activities and discussion questions:*

- If your breath sound assessment of a patient who complains of difficulty breathing is incorrect, how might that influence your concept formation?
- Why is knowledge of current evidence related to interpretation of clinical data important to clinical decision making?
- What factors can cause the decision making process to break down?

### *Summary assessment:*

- Administer the quiz related to this lesson (Evolve resources, instructor's test bank).

## ■ STUDY GUIDE ANSWERS

### EXERCISE 1 ■ *Case 15: 42-year-old male—difficulty breathing*

1. Below are the steps in the clinical decision-making process. What did you assess or do in each area (if anything) on this call, and what were your findings or actions?

| Elements of Decision Making | Steps in Process | Findings or Actions |
|---|---|---|
| Read the patient | Observe level of consciousness<br>Assess skin color and patient position<br>Determine chief complaint<br>Evaluate pulse<br>Auscultate lungs<br>Obtain vital signs | Awake and alert<br>Skin pale, cool clammy, seated<br>Difficulty breathing<br>Pulse irregular<br>Lungs clear<br>BP 106/68 mm Hg, P 120 bpm, R 36 breaths/min, $SaO_2$ 88% |
| Read the scene | Assess the general environment | Neat home, unremarkable; one family member present |

| Elements of Decision Making | Steps in Process | Findings or Actions |
|---|---|---|
| React | **Manage life threats when found** | **Apply oxygen** |
| Reevaluate | **Perform a focused or detailed assessment, or both** | **Neck: no JVD**<br>**Unremarkable** |
| Revise the treatment plan | **Revise treatment plan needed based on reevaluation** | **Continue oxygen; rapid transport** |
| Review performance at the run critique | **Perform both a formal or informal review** | **Review with instructor** |

*BP,* Blood pressure; *JVD,* jugular vein distension; *P,* pulse; *R,* respiration; *SaO₂,* oxygen saturation.

2. Why is it difficult to make a clear treatment decision on this patient?

**The picture does not quite fit anything that can be resolved in the prehospital setting. The patient has severe respiratory distress and low oxygen saturation, yet his lungs are clear and he does not have any life-threatening arrhythmia.**

3. What information helped your formation of the concept in this case?

**The chief complaint (difficulty breathing), general impression of the patient's level of distress, vital signs and physical examination, and history (long trip in a motor vehicle and cast recently removed) helped define the concept formation.**

4. Was there an algorithm or distinct treatment path that resolved this patient's crisis in the field? Explain your answer.

**No. This patient would be managed symptomatically and rapid transport to an appropriate facility performed.**

### EXERCISE 2 ■ *Case 2: 56-year-old female—fell*

5. What information on this call became barriers to the formation of your initial concept?

**The barriers included dispatch information that did not relate directly to the chief complaint, family member who was a poor historian, and a patient who was unable to provide detailed history because of critical condition.**

6. What features in the practice environment on this case increased the challenges of caring for this patient?

**The patient was found in a tight spot and would be difficult to access. She was on the floor, which would increase the difficulty in assessing her. The light is not optimal to evaluate her condition.**

7. When you viewed the initial video and had the information it presented, did you have sufficient data to place the patient's care into a standard treatment algorithm? Explain your answer.

**The information from the initial video did not provide sufficient information to initiate a plan of care. Although the patient needed supplemental oxygen, which was obvious from the video, further information was needed to proceed with additional care. Other information needed included breath sounds assessment, vital signs, oxygen saturation, ECG interpretation, and focused head-to-toe examination.**

# Assessment-Based Management

## ▪ Assignment

### Prerequisites:

- Complete Chapter 14, Assessment-Based Management, in *Mosby's Paramedic Textbook, Revised Third Edition*.
- Complete Chapter 14 in the workbook for *Mosby's Paramedic Textbook, Revised Third Edition*.
- Complete any skills or laboratory studies pertinent to this chapter.
- Read the "Getting Started" and "Orientation to Virtual Patient Encounters" sections in the *Virtual Patient Encounters Study Guide* (if this is the first lesson being attempted).

### Student assignment:

- Complete Lesson 14 in the *Virtual Patient Encounters Study Guide* after you have reviewed the topic in class.

## ▪ Topic Review

### Objectives:

*On completion of this lesson, the student will be able to perform the following:*

- Use *Pattern Recognition* to assess and treat each of the cases in this chapter.
- Form a field impression of the patient presented in each case, then develop and carry out a plan of action.

### Review the following topics with your students before they complete the lesson:

- To form a field impression, the paramedic must blend the elements of history and assessment with knowledge of pathophysiology, life-span development, and epidemiology.
- Pattern recognition forms the foundation to develop a field impression. Information gathered from the history and physical examination is compared with the paramedic's knowledge base of illness or injury to search for a diagnosis that fits a known pattern.
- Once the field impression has been determined, an action plan related to this impression is developed and implemented. Elements of the action plan will depend on the patient's condition and the environment.
- Treatment protocols or guidelines should guide the interventions in the action plan. This system may include basic and advanced life support measures.

- Factors that affect patient assessment and decision making include the paramedic's attitude, the patient's willingness to cooperate, distracting injuries, labeling or tunnel vision, environment, patient compliance, and personnel availability.

- Having an organized plan with predefined patient-care roles can minimize confusion and decrease mistakes. Roles can be assigned in a manner consistent with local operation protocols and available personnel. An example of team roles would be team leader and patient caregiver.

- Ensuring that the appropriate tools (or equipment) are readily available to assess and manage any given patient is also critical. Equipment bags vary by emergency medical services (EMS) systems and should enable the EMS crew to begin life-saving assessment and intervention without running back and forth to the ambulance.

- Two general approaches are applied to patient calls. The resuscitative approach is used when an immediate life threat exists. Immediate life-saving treatment is delivered before a complete history and physical are obtained. The contemplative approach is used when no imminent life threat is evident on arrival. In this approach, the history is taken, and a physical examination is performed before treatment is delivered.

- After assessment and care, information about the patient must be relayed to the receiving facility and then to the health care provider that will assume care of the patient. The report should be concise, free of jargon, follow a standard format, and present relevant findings and pertinent negatives.

## ■ Follow-Up

### *Assignment follow-up from previous class:*

- What problems, if any, did you have with your assignment?
- What questions do you have?

### *In-class activities and discussion questions:*

- Give the class some call dispatch information (play the actual calls if possible). Then, ask students what type of equipment they would bring in on the call. Based on the initial information from dispatch, have students predict whether the contemplative or resuscitative approach will be needed on the call.

- List three or four respiratory illnesses on the chalkboard. Have the class identify characteristics of each disease that would form a pattern to help them distinguish one from the other.

### *Summary assessment:*

- Administer the quiz related to this lesson (Evolve resources, instructor's test bank).

## ■ STUDY GUIDE ANSWERS

### EXERCISE 1 ■ *Case 1: 20-year-old male—difficulty breathing*

1. Has adequate information been provided by the resident advisor and firefighters to form a working field impression?

   **No, the paramedic must perform a brief physical examination in this case to include repeated vital signs, which may include pulse oximetry and capnography waveform assessment.**

2. What is your field impression of James' illness? Defend your answer.

**James is having an allergic reaction. This field impression is based on his history of an allergy to bee stings, his use of the EpiPen, and a history and physical examination that is characteristic for a patient having an allergic reaction.**

3. Is it possible that James may be suffering from more than one illness? What illness or illnesses do you suspect? Explain.

**James has history of asthma, which may make the allergic reaction worse for him. Asthma and an allergic reaction are both very similar, but in James' case a thorough physical examination reveals a swollen sting site on his leg.**

4. Based on your assessment and field impression, detail your action plan for James.

**Apply oxygen, gain intravenous access, repeat vital sign assessment every 5 minutes, and, if he is not improving, administer additional doses of epinephrine and consider administering diphenhydramine, inhaled beta agonists, and corticosteroids.**

## EXERCISE 2 ■ *Case 2: 56-year-old female—fell*

5. Does the woman's husband provide enough information to formulate a working field assessment?

**No, the paramedics must try to obtain more history information and complete a physical examination to include vital signs, an electrocardiogram (ECG) tracing, (12-lead ECG, if available).**

6. What attitude might the paramedic have to overcome to deal effectively with this patient?

**Society's impression of obesity**

7. What is your field impression of this patient?

**A cardiac event that may have caused her to become weak and fall**

8. Based on your assessment and field impression, detail your action plan for this patient.

**Apply high-flow oxygen. Gain intravenous access. Move the bedroom furniture to permit easy access to the patient. If her cervical spine or back is painful or injured, then maintain neutral alignment before moving her. With assistance, move her to the ambulance. Treat her for difficult breathing, chest pain, and weakness. Notify the receiving hospital of her impending arrival. Transport to a hospital with the appropriate cardiac care and bariatrics capabilities.**

## EXERCISE 3 ■ *Case 6: 16-year-old female—unknown medical*

9. What is your initial impression of this patient?

**Possible drug overdose or poisoning, altered consciousness or unconscious, and in need of a manual airway maneuver.**

10. What are your safety concerns about this patient?

**She may have suicide ideation, and a potential exists for blood or body fluid exposure.**

11. What is your field impression of this patient?

   **An unconscious female; possible medication overdose**

## EXERCISE 4 ■ *Case 7: 8-year-old male—submersion*

12. Would the initial approach to this patient change if he were still in the pool? Explain.

   **Yes. Removing him from the pool would be necessary using a long spine board and observing cervical spine precautions.**

13. What is your field impression of this patient?

   **An unconscious patient after a submersion or drowning incident, with possible head and cervical spine injuries**

14. Based on your field impression and initial assessment of this patient, detail your plan of action in order of importance.

   **Determine unresponsiveness, establish and maintain an airway and neutral alignment of the cervical spine using a jaw thrust maneuver, support the patient's respirations using the bag-mask device, move the patient onto a long spine board and secure him taking care to immobilize first the torso, then the head, initiate cardiac monitoring and gain intravenous access, evaluate the patient's respirations for advanced airway techniques and procedures, transport to an appropriate hospital.**

15. Where should this patient be transported? Explain.

   **The patient would ideally be transported to a pediatric trauma center because of his age and the nature of his injury.**

## EXERCISE 5 ■ *Case 8: 38-year-old male—suicide attempt*

16. What is your field impression of Robbie?

   **An altered mental status with delirium and possibly hallucinations**

17. What are some differential diagnoses for Robbie's behavior?

   **Hypoglycemia, hypoxia, substance abuse, head injury, stroke, brain tumors, and psychiatric disease**

18. How would your approach to Robbie change if the police officer had "tased" him?

   **He should be assessed now as an electrical injury because tasers deliver high voltage in short bursts and may interfere with normal cardiac conduction.**

19. Based on your field impression and assessment, detail a plan of action for Robbie.

   **Ensure your safety, as well as the safety of Bobbie, restrain Bobbie onto the cot on his back in four-point restraints, assess Bobbie to rule out other medical reasons for his behavior, and transport Bobbie to a hospital with mental health services.**

**EXERCISE 6** ■ *Case 12: 57-year-old male—man down*

20. What is your initial impression of Ted?

    **A sick man, possibly cardiac or diabetes related**

21. What extenuating circumstances need to be considered during your assessment?

    **Ted will need to be moved a considerable distance from the golf course to the waiting transport unit.**

22. Does Ted have risk factors for cardiac disease? If so, what are they?

    **Yes. Diabetes and hypertension; Ted is also obese.**

23. What are some differential diagnoses for Ted's signs and symptoms?

    **Heat-related illness, electrolyte imbalance, intoxication, cardiac arrhythmia, and complications of his diabetes**

# Communications

## ■ Assignment

### *Prerequisites:*

- Complete Chapter 15, Communications, in *Mosby's Paramedic Textbook, Revised Third Edition.*
- Complete Chapter 15 in the workbook for *Mosby's Paramedic Textbook, Revised Third Edition.*
- Complete any skills or laboratory studies pertinent to this lesson.
- Read the "Getting Started" and "Orientation to Virtual Patient Encounters" sections in the *Virtual Patient Encounters Study Guide* (if this is the first lesson being attempted).

### *Student assignment:*

- Complete Lesson 15 in the *Virtual Patient Encounters Study Guide* after you have reviewed the topic in class.

## ■ Topic Review

### *Objectives:*

*On completion of this lesson, the student will be able to perform the following:*

- Explain the importance of the dispatch information.
- Describe the effects of inadequate or inappropriate dispatch information.

### *Review the following topics with your students before they complete the lesson:*

- Five phases of communications occur during most emergency medical services (EMS) events:
    1. Occurrence of the event
    2. Detection of the need for EMS
    3. Notification and emergency response
    4. EMS arrival, treatment, and preparation for transport
    5. Preparation for the next response
- Proper verbal communication during an emergency event should be clear and brief and should follow local standards. Patient privacy should be protected.
- Dispatchers receive and process emergency calls, coordinate EMS resources, relay medical information, and coordinate with public safety agencies; their role is crucial.

- Emergency medical services dispatchers are trained to use guide cards or protocols, determine the nature of the call, determine the call priority, dispatch the appropriate equipment, and provide prearrival instructions to the caller when necessary.
- EMS communication protocols usually follow these guidelines:
  1. Think before you speak.
  2. Speak 2 to 3 inches from the microphone.
  3. Speak slowly, clearly, and in a normal pitch.
  4. Be brief.
  5. Avoid codes.
  6. Advise when your transmission is complete.
  7. Be professional.
- Patient information should be relayed to the receiving facility in a standard, concise format. Paramedic professionals should tell the hospital what they have found, what they have done, how the patient has responded, and when they will arrive.
- Errors in communication can result from attributes of the receiver, selective perception, semantic problems, and time pressures. Communication errors can have serious consequences related to scene safety, resource allocation, and patient care decision making.

## Follow-Up

### Assignment follow-up from previous class:

- What problems, if any, did you have with your assignment?
- What questions do you have?

### In-class activities and discussion questions:

- Ask the class to practice giving radio reports using walkie-talkie radios or tape recorders. Ask the other students to provide feedback regarding the effectiveness of the report.
- Play a version of the game *Telephone* during which you ask the class to stand in a circle then whisper a message to one student. Each student whispers the *same* message to the person beside him or her. The last student in the circle relates the message aloud. The final message is rarely exactly the same as the initial message.
- Discuss how communication failures occur and what measures can be taken to ensure consistent effective communication.

### Summary assessment:

- Administer the quiz related to this lesson (Evolve resources, instructor's test bank).

## STUDY GUIDE ANSWERS

### EXERCISE 1 ■ *Case 2: 56-year-old female—fell*

1. Did the dispatch complaint relate directly to the patient's chief complaint?

   **The dispatch information was for a fall. When the crew arrived on the call, the patient appeared to be ill with severe respiratory distress that resulted in a fall.**

2. Could the dispatch information affect what equipment these paramedics bring into the patient's home? Explain your answer.

   **The EMS crew, if given the incorrect dispatch information, might bring the wrong equipment into the home and fail to be prepared if the patient exhibits a life-threatening condition for which they are unprepared.**

3. Did the paramedics focus on the dispatch information as the chief cause of illness? Explain your answer.

   **No, the paramedic assessed the patient and tried to ascertain the true nature of her illness.**

4. How can incorrect dispatch information delay the response to the scene?

   **If the dispatch information leads a crew to believe that no life threat exists, then district protocols may indicate a nonemergency response (no lights and sirens). In some circumstances, this status can cause a delay in the response time to the call.**

5. After the paramedic spoke with the patient's husband, what information should he have communicated to his partner?

   **He should communicate the relevant information about the patient's medical history and let his partner know what medications the patient is taking.**

**EXERCISE 2 ■ *Case 7: 8-year-old male—submersion***
**                          *Case 11: 32-year-old male—gunshot wounds***

6. What effect could incorrect dispatch information have had in each of these cases?
   a. Case 7:

      **Incorrect information can result in improper equipment arriving at the patient's side in a timely manner. For example, if the crew did not know the patient was a child, then they may not have brought age-appropriate supplies. If the crew did not know the call was related to a drowning, then they may not have brought supplies to provide spinal motion restriction to the patient or had suction readily available.**

   b. Case 11:

      **In this case, without proper information, the crew may not have worn appropriate personal protective equipment to approach the scene. They may not have known whether the scene was safe or if a need existed to stage an appropriate distance from the scene until it was cleared by police.**

7. If the dispatch information sounds odd to you, then what should you do in each of these cases?

   **If something sounds incorrect about a dispatch —the wrong address or unusual information— then contacting dispatch for additional information would be appropriate.**

# Documentation

## ■ Assignment

### Prerequisites:

- Complete Chapter 16, Documentation, in *Mosby's Paramedic Textbook, Revised Third Edition.*
- Complete Chapter 16 in the workbook for *Mosby's Paramedic Textbook, Revised Third Edition.*
- Complete any skills or laboratory studies pertinent to this chapter.
- Read the "Getting Started" and "Orientation to Virtual Patient Encounters" sections in the *Virtual Patient Encounters Study Guide* (if this is the first lesson being attempted).

### Student assignment:

- Complete Lesson 16 in the *Virtual Patient Encounters Study Guide* after you have reviewed the topic in class.

## ■ Topic Review

### Objectives:

*On completion of this lesson, the student will be able to perform the following:*

- Identify and document important information that should be included in your patient care report from a scene size-up.
- Choose the best format from different reporting styles for various patients with different types of medical and trauma conditions.
- Accurately and completely document subjective and objective findings from dispatch through various points in patient interactions, including initial assessment and interventions, as well as the rapid physical examination.
- Identify and apply reporting strategies you would use in special circumstances such as when a crime may be involved.
- Demonstrate how you would document patient response to the delivery of incorrect care.

### Review the following topics with your students before they complete the lesson:

- The patient care report is used to document patient assessment, care, and transport.
- The patient care report should be legible; slang should be avoided; only approved abbreviations should be used; dates and times should be included; and any difficulties encountered, previous care that was provided, and occurrences and interventions should be noted.

- Times that should be documented include time of call, dispatch, arrival at scene, arrival at patient, vital sign assessment, interventions, departure from scene, arrival at medical facility, and return to service.
- The narrative is the chronologic account of the call. It should include pertinent negative findings and pertinent statements.
- A well-written report should be accurate and complete, legible, timely, unaltered, and free of non-professional or extraneous information.
- Narrative formats include the SOAP format, the CHART format, the physical approach from head-to-toe, a review of primary body systems, or a chronologic, call-incident approach.
- SOAP format stands for Subjective data, Objective data, Assessment data, and Plan of patient management.
- CHART format stands for Chief complaint, History, Assessment, Rx (treatment), and Transport.

## Follow-Up

### Assignment follow-up from previous class:

- What problems, if any, did you have with your assignment?
- What questions do you have?

### In-class activities and discussion questions:

- What is the advantage of adopting a consistent method to document patient information?
- How will accurate, clear, and complete documentation help you if you are called to testify in court?

### Summary assessment:

- Administer the quiz related to this lesson (Evolve resources, instructor's test bank).

## STUDY GUIDE ANSWERS

### EXERCISE 1 ■ Case 1: 20-year-old male—difficulty breathing

1. Begin the narrative in the following table using the CHART format. Provide the following information:

| Aspect to Document | Answer |
| --- | --- |
| Chief complaint | **Difficulty breathing** |
| History | **Should include history of allergies, reported event, and treatments administered before arrival and results** |
| Assessment | **Should include general impression, audible respirations before seeing patient, observations of position, use of accessory muscles, two-word dyspnea, findings from the Look, Listen, and Feel buttons—skin color and temperature, wheezes—observable site of sting, and vital signs or a notation to note vital signs as listed in the vital sign area** |

**EXERCISE 2 ■** *Case 11: 32-year-old male—gunshot wounds*

2. Before you start the case, consider what you might observe at the scene of a crime that involves a gunshot that would be considered important and should be included in the patient care report. List three observations.

   **Possible answers include the following: (a) type of gun present, (b) spent shells present, and (c) amount of blood present. Additional answers include blood proximity to patient location, numbers of victims, and treatments being provided by law enforcement.**

3. Using the chronologic call-incident approach, write the first few sentences that would appear in your patient care narrative for this patient.

   **Ambulance 41 was dispatched to 104 Charles St for a report of shots fired. On arrival, met by police, who reported that a 32-year-old male had been shot three times at close range. The patient was located on the front porch, supine, with blood visible in several places on the right side of his shirt. Patient was unresponsive to verbal stimulus or touch. Manual spinal stabilization applied, airway maintained, and breathing and carotid pulse assessed and present.**

4. Describe how you would document the locations of the apparent bullet wounds you observed after opening the shirt.

   **On examination, noted three apparent bullet wounds, one in the lateral right upper quadrant, one in the right upper chest, approximately 1 inch inferior of the clavicle in the mid-clavicular line and one to right lateral neck.**

5. Using the information gained, add these objective findings as you would document them in the narrative and vital signs areas in a patient care report.

   **Patient has gasping respirations with abdominal breathing present and using accessory neck muscles; left lung sounds present and clear; absent right. Pulse present and weak. Skin pale, cool, and diaphoretic above clavicles and dry below. Abdomen rigid. All four extremities cool and diaphoretic; no movement present. Vital sign area would indicate respirations 8, pulse 128 and regular, and BP 82/56 regular.**

**EXERCISE 3 ■** *Case 9: 22-year-old female—assault*

6. Recognizing that this case will likely go to court and that your patient care report will be evidence, consider what general observations about the patient's environment might be important and should be included in the patient care report. List two observations.

   **The condition of the environment might include the following: (a) overturned furniture and (b) broken objects. Additional observations include the presence and proximity of objects that may have been used to assault the patient if the assault occurred at that location.**

7. List several observations you would include on your report that would describe the apparent psychologic state of the patient with the expectation that you will present these observations in court.

   **Demeanor, posture, position, and stance; diverted gaze; fingers clenched; voice shaky, trembling, and sounding frightened**

8. You decide to perform a limited physical examination of the patient. How would your patient care report indicate the fact that you did not conduct a physical examination of the patient specific to the sexual assault?

**The report could indicate that the genital examination was deferred. Report that no bleeding is reported by the patient.**

### EXERCISE 4 ■ *Case 14: 65-year-old male—difficulty breathing*

9. This patient, when asked what was wrong, responded with two complaints. Which method of narrative reporting, SOAP or CHART, would work best in this case? Explain your answer.

**The SOAP method would seem to be a better choice because this patient has already given the paramedic two important pieces of subjective information in response to this question. The CHART method will work better when one clear chief complaint exists, although many EMS personnel choose one method to document calls so their documentation will be consistent.**

10. Complete the first part of your narrative using the SOAP format. List all the subjective data, skip a line, and then list all the objective data.

**Subjective: 10/10 dyspnea worsening over 2 days and preventing sleep, nonradiating chest pain, orthopnea, nausea, weak, and tired**

**Objective: Tripoding, two- to four-word dyspnea, diaphoretic, pedal edema, and wet cough**

### EXERCISE 5 ■ *Case 13: 5-month-old male—unresponsive*

11. Keeping in mind that the parent has not accompanied you, what method of reporting will likely work best with this patient—SOAP, CHART, or the chronologic call-incident approach? Explain why your choice would be the best.

**The chronologic, call-incident approach is the best choice for this call, given that extremely limited historical information is available and because many interventions can be initiated with this patient. Many EMS providers choose one method to document calls so that their documentation will be consistent.**

12. Begin your report using the chronologic call-incident approach, beginning with your dispatch and continuing through the application of CPR using basic life support equipment.

**The report should include findings and observations that include absence of pulse and respiration, appearance of all body areas (look), and findings of all body areas as noted with feel, method of opening the airway, inability to insert oropharyngeal airway until suction performed, ventilation via bag-valve-mask with correct oxygen flow, and application of CPR.**

**EXERCISE 6 ■ *Case 8: 38-year-old male—suicide attempt***

13. The police have secured this patient on a stretcher. You will need to document this restraint in your patient care report. List the appropriate dispatch information and your initial observations of the patient in a manner that justifies your decision to allow the police to gain control of the patient.

**You were dispatched for a suicide attempt. You should describe the danger of the physical location of the patient, the physical actions and movements of the patient, and the general flow and content of the patient's verbal statements. Also document your actions to immediately reposition the patient so he is not prone.**

14. Because the police had to use force with this patient, some physical injuries may have resulted. Indicate how you would document the capture, restraint, and move of the patient to the stretcher by the police.

**The report should include how the patient was captured while running away, moved face down to the ground, handcuffed behind his back, legs tied or hog tied, and carried and placed face down on the stretcher. If any trauma to the patient was noted when you assumed his care, document it.**

15. Describe how you would document the initial actions you take after the police have positioned the patient on the stretcher and prepared him for transportation, including the actions you would take to reposition the patient appropriately.

**The patient is placed prone on a stretcher by the police with the patient's arms handcuffed behind his back. The handcuffs are then removed, extremities are manually restrained, and the patient is rolled supine (or lateral). The patient's extremities are secured to the ambulance cot using soft restraints (or leather restraints). One arm is restrained above the patient's head to the side of the cot, and the other arm is restrained to the patient's side. The patient is reevaluated after being restrained. The airway is patent; the capillary refill is less than 2 seconds in all extremities; and his distal extremities are pink, warm, and dry. The patient remains agitated; however, he does not verbalize any pain as a result of the restraint. Continual end-tidal $CO_2$ and visual monitoring of the patient are performed.**

# Pharmacology

## ■ Assignment

### Prerequisites:

- Complete Chapter 17, Pharmacology, in *Mosby's Paramedic Textbook, Revised Third Edition*.
- Complete Chapter 17 in the workbook for *Mosby's Paramedic Textbook, Revised Third Edition*.
- Complete any skills or laboratory studies pertinent to this chapter.
- Read the "Getting Started" and "Orientation to Virtual Patient Encounters" sections in the *Virtual Patient Encounters Study Guide* (if this is the first lesson being attempted).

### Student assignment:

- Complete Lesson 17 in the *Virtual Patient Encounters Study Guide* after you have reviewed the topic in class.

## ■ Topic Review

### Objectives:

*On completion of this lesson, the student will be able to perform the following:*

- Recognize the role of medication identification in determining the clinical impression.
- Distinguish onset, peak, and duration of action of various types of insulin.
- Outline the actions of various types of antihypertensive medications.
- Value the importance of interpreting patient medication therapy as part of the assessment process.
- Be familiar with the profiles of commonly prescribed medications.

### Review the following topics with your students before they complete the lesson:

- The paramedic must have a detailed understanding of the drugs that are administered in the pre-hospital setting. Equally important, the paramedic must recognize the medications that the patient is taking at home. This knowledge will help you form a field diagnosis and make appropriate treatment decisions.
- The action of drugs is influenced by the patient's age, body mass, gender, environment, time of administration, pathologic state, and genetic and psychologic factors.
- The drug dose that produces the desired effect without causing harm is the therapeutic range.
- The biologic half-life is the time to metabolize one-half of the drug. The longer the half-life is, the longer the drug will exert its action in the body.

- The therapeutic index measures the relative safety of a drug, which is the ratio between the dose that is lethal in 50% of patients and the dose that is effective in 50% of patients. The closer the ratio is to 1 is, the more likely the drug will cause undesirable effects.
- Special indications, contraindication, or dose modifications may exist that need to be made for certain patient groups. These groups include children, older adults, and pregnant patients.

# ■ Follow-Up

### *Assignment follow-up from previous class:*

- What problems, if any, did you have with your assignment?
- What questions do you have?

### *In-class activities and discussion questions:*

- Assemble a collection of actual prescription medication bottles from family and colleagues. Divide the class into small groups and give students several medication bottles. Ask students to predict (1) what illness a patient might have based on the medication and (2) if this medicine would influence their patient care.
- Have students use a pocket guide, such as *Rapid Paramedic, Revised Edition*, to assist with the task.
- Discuss why portable resources such as this one are essential tools for the paramedic.

### *Summary assessment:*

- Administer the quiz related to this lesson (Evolve resources, instructor's test bank).

# ■ STUDY GUIDE ANSWERS

### EXERCISE 1 ■ *Case 2: 56-year-old female—fell*

1. What historical information missing on the call could have assisted you in making a clinical decision?

   **The patient and her husband were vague about her medical history. When asked about the medications that his wife takes, he handed the crew a box of medicines.**

2. Assuming that this patient's husband gave the paramedic the medications listed in each of the following examples, find each of the drugs in the "Emergency Drug Index" at the back of your text, in the "Drug Guide" in the software, or in Mosby's *Essential Drug List for Mosby's Paramedic Textbook* on Evolve (http://evolve.elsevier.com/Sanders/paramedic). Then identify the class of the drug and what conditions each drug is used to treat. Finally, under "Impression," list some possible causes of the patient's difficulty breathing, based on this information.

   **EXAMPLE 1** (same medications as listed in the history in software)

   | Medications | Drug Class | Medicines Prescribed for |
   | --- | --- | --- |
   | Lanoxin | **Cardiac glycoside** | **Congestive heart failure, tachycardias** |
   | Bumex | **Loop diuretic** | **Hypertension, congestive heart failure** |

**EXAMPLE 1**—*Continued*

| Medications | Drug Class | Medicines Prescribed for |
|---|---|---|
| Hydrochlorothiazide | Thiazide diuretic | Hypertension |
| Serevent | Beta-2 agonist | Bronchoconstriction associated with asthma and chronic obstructive pulmonary disease |
| Albuterol | Beta-2 agonist | Bronchoconstriction associated with asthma or chronic obstructive pulmonary disease |

Impression: **Exacerbation of congestive heart failure, chronic obstructive pulmonary disease, or spontaneous pneumothorax secondary to ruptured bleb**

**EXAMPLE 2**

| Medications | Drug Class | Medicines Prescribed for |
|---|---|---|
| Coreg | Beta-blocker | Hypertension, congestive heart failure |
| Spironolactone | Potassium-sparing diuretic | Hypertension, congestive heart failure |
| Diovan | Angiotensin II receptor antagonist | Hypertension, congestive heart failure |
| Furosemide | Loop diuretic | Hypertension, edema |

Impression: **Hypertension, congestive heart failure**

**EXAMPLE 3**

| Medications | Drug Class | Medicines Prescribed for |
|---|---|---|
| Rifampin | Antitubercular agent | Treat infections: tuberculosis, staphylococcus infection, meningitis |
| Isoniazid | Antitubercular agent | Tuberculosis |
| Combivent | Antitubercular agent | Bronchodilator |

Impression: **Tuberculosis**

## EXAMPLE 4

| Medications | Drug Class | Medicines Prescribed for |
|---|---|---|
| Singulair | Leukotriene receptor antagonist | Used to prevent bronchoconstriction related to asthma, chronic obstructive pulmonary disease |
| Maxair | Beta-2 agonist | Relieves bronchospasm |
| Advair | Steroid and long-acting bronchodilator | Bronchodilation |

Impression: **Asthma or chronic obstructive pulmonary disease**

## EXAMPLE 5

| Medications | Drug Class | Medicines Prescribed for |
|---|---|---|
| Isosorbide | Vasodilator | Angina |
| Persantine | Antiplatelet | Prevents clotting |
| Lipitor | Statin | Lowers cholesterol |
| Accupril | Angiotensin-converting enzyme (ACE) inhibitor | Hypertension, lowers risk of acute coronary syndrome |

Impression: **At risk for ST-segment elevation myocardial infarction, cardiac history, possible congestive heart failure**

## EXAMPLE 6

| Medications | Drug Class | Medicines Prescribed for |
|---|---|---|
| Combivir | Antiviral | Human immunodeficiency virus (HIV) |
| Indinavir (Crixivan) | Protease inhibitor | HIV |

Impression: **Pneumonia or other complication related to HIV is possible or heart disease**

## EXAMPLE 7

| Medications | Drug Class | Medicines Prescribed for |
|---|---|---|
| Metformin | | Diabetes |
| Avalide | | Diabetes |
| Repaglinide (Prandin) | | Diabetes |

Impression: **High risk for heart disease because of diabetes**

## EXERCISE 2 ■ *Case 4: 64-year-old male—unknown medical*

3. You find a medication list on this patient's refrigerator that indicates he is taking insulin. Fill in the missing information related to the generic or trade name, and then list how long it takes to achieve the peak effect and the duration of effect of each of the following insulins when administered subcutaneously.

| Generic Name | Trade Name | Onset of Effect | Peak Effect | Duration |
|---|---|---|---|---|
| **Insulin zinc suspension recombinant human** | Humulin U | 4-8 hr | 8-20 hr | 24-48 hr |
| Insulin recombinant human | **Humulin R Velosulin BR Novulin R** | 30-60 min | 1-5 hr | 6-10 hr |
| **Insulin glargine recombinant** | Lantus | 1 hr | 5 hr | 25 hr |
| Insulin aspart recombinant | **NovoLog** | 15 min | 1-3 hr | 3-5 hr |
| **Insulin glulisine** | Apidra | 15 min | 0.5-1.5 hr | 1.0-2.5 hr |

4. Which of the insulins listed in the previous table may be given by insulin pump?
   **Insulin glulisine can be given by insulin pump.**

5. Why is it important to know the time of onset, peak action, and duration for each insulin?
   **Knowing the time of onset, peak action, and duration can help to determine if this patient's response is predictable or if another coexisting problem exists. In addition, understanding this information is important so you can provide the patient with appropriate education to prevent the occurrence of hypoglycemia.**

## EXERCISE 3 ■ *Case 12: 57-year-old male—man down*

6. The patient in this case is taking two antihypertensive agents, Vasotec and Bumex. Many types of drugs are used to treat hypertension. Complete the information in the following table related to these and other antihypertensive agents.

| Generic Name | Trade Name | Drug Classification | Action |
|---|---|---|---|
| doxazosin | **Cardura** | **Alpha-1 receptor blocker** | **Causes vasodilation by inhibiting the alpha-1 sympathetic effect on the arteries.** |
| **enalapril** | Vasotec | **Angiotensin-converting enzyme (ACE) inhibitor** | **Prevents conversion of angiotension I to angiotension II in the lungs. Angiotension II is a potent vasoconstrictor.** |

| Generic Name | Trade Name | Drug Classification | Action |
|---|---|---|---|
| irbesartan | **Avapro** | **Angiotensin-receptor blocker** | **Prevents the vasoconstriction effects of angiotensin at the arterial receptors.** |
| **metoprolol long-acting** | Toprol XL | **Beta-adrenergic–blocking agent** | **Decreases heart rate and contractility.** |
| amlidopine | **Norvasc** | **Calcium channel blocker** | **Causes arteriolar vasodilation.** |
| **bumetanide** | Bumex | **Loop diuretic; antihypertensive** | **Inhibits sodium reabsorption in ascending limb of the loop of Henle.** |
| **hydrochlorothiazide** | Hydrodiuril | **Thiazide diuretic; antihypertensive** | **Affects reabsorption of electrolytes in distal renal tubules.** |

## EXERCISE 4 ■ *Case 5: 40-year-old male—vomiting blood*

7. Describe how this patient's present illness and medical history will affect drug absorption, distribution, and biotransformation and how these could affect drug therapy if it were indicated.

| | Absorption | Distribution | Biotransformation |
|---|---|---|---|
| Illness effects on each | **Patient is hypotensive; thus drugs given by routes other than intravenously will be absorbed slowly.** | **Distribution will be slowed because of poor perfusion. Plasma protein may be decreased in this patient if he has liver disease from chronic alcoholism. This condition will lower binding sites for plasma-bound drugs.** | **Orally administered drugs are metabolized in the liver before they enter the general circulation. This action reduces the amount of active drug to circulate to the tissues. If this patient's liver function is impaired, then higher-than-expected drug levels may occur when drugs are given enterally.** |
| Impact of drug treatment (if indicated) | **Avoid oral, intramuscular, or subcutaneous drug routes until perfusion improves.** | **May take longer for drug effects to appear. Dosing may need to be altered in some cases.** | **Oral drug doses may need to be adjusted.** |

# Venous Access and Medication Administration

## ■ Assignment

### Prerequisites:

- Complete Chapter 18, Venous Access and Medication Administration, in *Mosby's Paramedic Textbook, Revised Third Edition*.
- Complete Chapter 18 in the workbook for *Mosby's Paramedic Textbook, Revised Third Edition*.
- Complete any skills or laboratory studies pertinent to this chapter.
- Read the "Getting Started" and "Orientation to Virtual Patient Encounters" sections in the *Virtual Patient Encounters Study Guide* (if this is the first lesson being attempted).

### Student assignment:

- Complete Lesson 18 in the *Virtual Patient Encounters Study Guide* after you have reviewed the topic in class.

## ■ Topic Review

### Objectives:

*On completion of this lesson, the student will be able to perform the following:*

- Determine appropriate situations for the use of intraosseous infusion.
- Identify appropriate medication administration routes based on an understanding of lifespan development.
- Calculate drug doses accurately.

### Review the following topics with your students before they complete the lesson:

- To deliver appropriate advanced life support care, paramedics must be able to administer prescribed medications and initiate vascular access.
- Several drug calculation methods can be used. You should select the one with which you are most comfortable and use it consistently so you can calculate drug doses accurately in the most stressful situations.
- When administering drugs to patients, use the following safe practices: Avoid distractions, repeat orders to ensure you clearly understand them, confirm the information on the drug label at least three times, use the correct route of administration, avoid giving medication from an unlabeled container, confirm calculations if you are unsure, use aseptic technique with multidose vials, label a syringe if you do not administer the drug immediately, check expiration dates, double check if someone questions the drug or dose, monitor the patient for adverse effects, document, and dispose of unused medicine appropriately.

- Medication administration in the prehospital setting is given by the oral, transdermal, rectal, sublingual, subcutaneous, intramuscular, intravenous, intraosseous, intranasal, and endotracheal routes.
- Subcutaneous medication administration is a parenteral route of medication administration that provides slower absorption and therefore more sustained action of drugs. The drug is injected into the subcutaneous fat when given by this route.
- Intramuscular medication administration is used for faster absorption than subcutaneous administration. The intramuscular route permits more sustained action than the intravenous route. Several muscles are used for intramuscular administration, including the deltoid, dorsogluteal, and vastus lateralis sites. You must select the appropriate site based on the volume and type of drug to be given and the accessibility of the site.
- If vascular access is not possible and a life-threatening condition exists that requires administration of medication or fluids, then the intraosseous site should be considered. Newer access devices have made this route accessible in adults and children. Once access is established, the same medication and fluids administered by intravascular access can be given through this site.

## ■ Follow-Up

### *Assignment follow-up from previous class:*

- What problems, if any, did you have with your assignment?
- What questions do you have?

### *In-class activities and discussion questions:*

- Give students four or five drug dose calculation problems. Have students write their answers anonymously to the problem on a blank sheet of paper. Select several incorrect doses, and have the class discuss the possible effects of overdosing or underdosing this medication.
- Divide the class into groups. Give each group several case studies with a desired drug dose to be administered. Provide the actual drug container, and have students calculate the number of milliliters to be administered. Then, have students draw up the correct volume of medicine.

### *Summary assessment:*

- Administer the quiz related to this lesson (Evolve resources, instructor's test bank).

## ■ STUDY GUIDE ANSWERS

**EXERCISE 1** ■ *Case 5: 40-year-old male—vomiting blood*
*Case 13: 5-month-old male—unresponsive*

1. Would the intraosseous route be an acceptable vascular access route in each of these cases?
   a. Case 5:

   **Intraosseous would be an appropriate vascular access device if the proper equipment were available for access.**

   b. Case 13:

   **Intraosseous vascular access would be appropriate for this infant.**

2. At what point would you elect to perform intraosseous access in each of these cases?

   a. Case 5:

      **If other efforts to establish peripheral access are not successful and the patient's condition is critical, then you might attempt to establish intraosseous access (according to your local protocol).**

   b. Case 13:

      **If vascular access cannot be established immediately in an infant in cardiac arrest, then intraosseous access should be attempted.**

3. Why is the intraosseous route preferred over the endotracheal route?

   **Absorption is unpredictable when drugs are given by the endotracheal route; thus vascular access—intravenous or intraosseous—is preferred.**

4. In each of the two cases (assuming the patient has a pulse and is perfusing well), describe an appropriate site for administration of an intramuscular injection.

   a. Case 5:

      **Intramuscular injection might be given to this patient in his deltoid muscle or in the vastus lateralis muscle if he is supine.**

   b. Case 13:

      **Intramuscular injection should be given in the vastus lateralis muscle in infants of this age.**

5. Assume you want to administer dopamine 5 mcg/kg/min. You have 200 mg dopamine in 250 ml $D_5W$. Your IV tubing drop factor is 60 gtt/ml. How many drops per minute will you run your fluid?

   a. Case 5:

      **32 gtt/min**

   b. Case 13:

      **3 gtt/min**

6. Assume you want to administer lidocaine 2 mg/min to the patient in Case 5. You have 1 g lidocaine in 250 ml $D_5W$. Your IV tubing drop factor is 60 gtt/ml. How many drops per minute will you run your fluid?

   **30 gtt/min**

7. Assume you want to administer a 20 ml/kg fluid bolus over 20 minutes to the patient in Case 13. Your IV tubing drop factor is 20 gtt/ml. How many drops per minute will you run your fluid?

   **145 gtt/min**

### EXERCISE 2 ■ *Case 12: 57-year-old male—man down*

8. Assume that you determined the patient needed the following drugs and dosing schedule after you completed your history and physical examination and determined your diagnosis. Identify the proper route of administration, then calculate the correct volume or drip rate to administer. Assume that the macrodrip IV tubing delivers 10 gtt/ml.

| Condition | Drug or Dose | Route | Volume (or gtt/min) to Administer |
|---|---|---|---|
| Dehydration | Normal saline 250 ml over 20 min | IV infusion | 125 gtt/min |
| Hypoglycemia | 25 g 50% Dextrose | IV infusion | 25 ml |
| OxyContin overdose | Naloxone 0.8 mg IV (supplied as 2 mg in 2 ml) | IV, IM, SQ, IN, ET | 0.8 ml |
| Nausea and vomiting | Promethazine 12.5 mg (supplied as 50 mg/ml) | IV or deep IM | 0.25 ml |

*IM,* Intramuscular; *IN,* intranasal; *IV,* intravenous.

# Airway Management and Ventilation

## ■ Assignment

### *Prerequisites:*

- Complete Chapter 19, Airway Management and Ventilation, in *Mosby's Paramedic Textbook, Revised Third Edition*.
- Complete Chapter 19 in the workbook for *Mosby's Paramedic Textbook, Revised Third Edition*.
- Complete any skills or laboratory studies pertinent to this lesson.
- Read the "Getting Started" and "Orientation to Virtual Patient Encounters" sections in the *Virtual Patient Encounters Study Guide* (if this is the first lesson being attempted).

### *Student assignment:*

- Complete Lesson 19 in the *Virtual Patient Encounters Study Guide* after you have reviewed the topic in class.

## ■ Topic Review

### *Objectives:*

*On completion of this lesson, the student will be able to perform the following:*

- Assess and manage an airway obstruction.
- Use preventive measures for pulmonary aspiration.
- Evaluate airway for patency and breathing for adequacy.

### *Review the following topics with your students before they complete the lesson:*

- The absence of adequate airway and ineffective ventilation are major causes of preventable death and cardiopulmonary complications in all patients.
- External respiration is the transfer of oxygen and carbon dioxide between the inspired air and pulmonary capillaries. Internal respiration is the transfer of oxygen and carbon dioxide between the capillary red blood cells and tissue cells. Any disease or illness that interferes with either phase can cause hypoxia.
- Immediate assessment and management of airway, ventilation, and oxygenation take priority over all other patient care efforts. Specialized tools to assess the airway include pulse oximetry and capnography.

- If the patient is unconscious and cervical spine trauma is not indicated, open the airway using the head-tilt/chin-lift maneuver. Then, look for chest rise and fall, and listen and feel for air movement. If the patient is not breathing, assist ventilation and insert an oropharyngeal or nasopharyngeal airway. Insert an advanced airway when possible.
- If the patient is breathing, assess for the quality and adequacy of ventilation. Determine the rate, quality, and regularity of breathing. Inspect for accessory muscle use. Deliver oxygen therapy based on the breathing assessment and the patient's underlying condition. Assist ventilation if it is inadequate.
- Pulse oximetry can assist in evaluating whether the patient is receiving adequate oxygenation. Some conditions can create a false impression that the patient is well oxygenated. These conditions include carbon monoxide poisoning and methemoglobinemia. Changes in oximetry will not immediately occur when the patient's ventilatory status changes—they take minutes.
- Capnography is a measurement of ventilation. The shape of the waveform may quickly provide information related to apnea, endotracheal tube displacement, and bronchospasm. Changes in the patient's ventilation status will be immediately observed on the capnographic waveform. The adequacy of spontaneous or assisted ventilation can be evaluated using capnography. Normal end-tidal carbon dioxide ($EtCO_2$) is 35 to 45 mm Hg.
- $EtCO_2$ will be elevated when ventilation is decreased or when $CO_2$ production is increased.
- Low $EtCO_2$ readings may be found if a ventilation problem develops, if blood flow is inadequate, if ventilation perfusion is mismatched or production of $CO_2$ is decreased, if the tubing is blocked, or if a sampling error has developed.

## ◼ Follow-Up

### Assignment follow-up from previous class:

- What problems, if any, did you have with your assignment?
- What questions do you have?

### In-class activities and discussion questions:

- List some specific clinical case examples in which a patient would be expected to have an increase in $EtCO_2$ levels.
- What is the clinical significance of identifying a shark fin waveform on the $EtCO_2$ monitor?
- Explain why clinical methods alone are not sufficient to confirm correct placement of an endotracheal tube.

### Summary assessment:

- Administer the quiz related to this lesson (Evolve resources, instructor's test bank).

## ◼ STUDY GUIDE ANSWERS

### EXERCISE 1 ◼ Preparation Activity

1. What conditions or diseases might reduce oxygen available for exchange at the alveolar level?

   **Airway obstructions, low oxygen atmosphere such as a trench, chemical spill, or carbon monoxide–rich environment**

2. List ways in which a patient might be treated for low oxygen levels.

   **Relieve airway obstructions, apply supplemental oxygen, and remove the patient from any hazardous environment.**

3. What conditions or diseases impair circulation of red blood cells to the tissue?

   **Shock states such as hypovolemia, cardiac-related shock, peripheral vasodilation associated with spine injury**

4. List ways in which a patient might be treated for impaired circulation.

   **Cardiopulmonary resuscitation, fluid resuscitation, use of pressor agents**

5. What conditions or diseases impair the exchange of oxygen and carbon dioxide at the alveolar level and again at the cellular level?

   **Chronic obstructive pulmonary disease, tension pneumothorax, pneumonia, chest trauma, pulmonary contusions**

6. List ways in which a patient might be treated for impaired oxygen–carbon dioxide exchange.

   **Apply supplemental oxygen; ventilate the patient with the bag-mask device and supplemental oxygen, needle decompression thoracotomy, advanced airway devices.**

## EXERCISE 2 ■ Case 1: 20-year-old male—difficulty breathing

7. What is causing James' difficulty breathing?

   **Laryngeal spasm or edema, and bronchospasm**

8. What would the benefit be for James if oxygen were applied?

   **Decreased inspiratory volumes will result in decreased oxygen available to be used at the alveolar level; therefore increasing oxygen concentration available in inspired air would make more oxygen available at the alveolar level.**

9. Did pulse oximetry provide useful information in this case? Why or why not?

   **Yes, the oxygen saturation value will guide the paramedic toward more effective treatments or stopping treatments when improvements are noted.**

10. Would capnography provide useful information in this case? Why or why not?

    **Yes, capnographic waveforms will assist the paramedic in evaluating James' ventilation.**

## EXERCISE 3 ■ Case 2: 56-year-old female—fell

11. List the signs of respiratory distress that you observe in this patient.

    **Tachypnea, diaphoresis, difficulty speaking**

12. The original dispatch was for a woman who fell. List possible causes of her dyspnea.

    **One or more broken ribs, pulmonary contusion, pulmonary embolism, allergic reaction, congestive heart failure**

13. List physiologic concerns that may make management of this patient's airway, oxygenation, and ventilation more difficult.

**The patient is obese; therefore advanced airway procedures and bag-mask ventilation will be more difficult. She will most likely be more comfortable in a head-up position.**

14. Did pulse oximetry provide valuable information in this patient? Why or why not?

**No, she is hypotensive.**

15. Did capnography provide valuable information in this patient? Why or why not?

**Yes, it would permit the paramedic to measure and evaluate ventilation in this patient.**

## EXERCISE 4 ■ *Case 5: 40-year-old male—vomiting blood*

16. Before beginning the video, review the steps for suctioning on pages 466 through 468 of your textbook and list below.

**Preoxygenate the patient, pass the suction catheter or rigid tip device into the oropharynx without suction being applied, withdraw the suction catheter or rigid device with suction applied, and oxygenate the patient and evaluate the respiratory status.**

17. What concerns do you have about this patient's airway?

**He may vomit and aspirate the vomitus, especially given that he has been drinking and may be impaired.**

18. How would you prepare yourself to care for this patient's airway?

**Prepare the suction device and keep it close by in case he vomits. Consider transporting the patient in a left lateral recumbent position. Oxygen should probably be administered via nasal cannula.**

19. Did pulse oximetry provide useful information in this case? Why or why not?

**Most likely not; his blood pressure is too low.**

20. Would capnography provide useful information in this case? Why or why not?

**Frequent vomiting could interfere with collecting breath samples, it would depend on the type of EtCO$_2$ monitoring device.**

## EXERCISE 5 ■ *Case 6: 16-year-old female—unknown medical*

21. Before beginning the video, review the steps for insertion of the nasopharyngeal airway on pages 469 to 471 of your textbook and list below.

**Select the proper sized device (18 to 21 French for this case), lubricate the device with a water soluble lubricant, place the device into the nostril with the bevel directed toward the septum, pass the device gently into the nose taking care not to force it, reevaluate the patient's respiratory status.**

22. What are your management priorities for Sarah?

    **Position Sarah's head to maintain her airway, secure a patent airway, protect the airway and prepare for vomiting, provide ventilatory support as needed, provide high-flow oxygen, evaluate Sarah for more advanced airway techniques.**

23. Would pulse oximetry provide valuable information on Sarah? Why or why not?

    **Most likely not; her blood pressure is too low.**

24. Would capnography provide valuable information on Sarah? Why or why not?

    **Yes, capnography might be used to monitor hypoventilation.**

# Trauma Systems and Mechanism of Injury

## ▪ Assignment

### *Prerequisites:*

- Complete Chapter 20, Trauma Systems and Mechanism of Injury, in *Mosby's Paramedic Textbook, Revised Third Edition.*
- Complete Chapter 20 in the workbook for *Mosby's Paramedic Textbook, Revised Third Edition.*
- Complete any skills or laboratory studies pertinent to this chapter.
- Read the "Getting Started" and "Orientation to Virtual Patient Encounters" sections in the *Virtual Patient Encounters Study Guide* (if this is the first lesson being attempted).

### *Student assignment:*

- Complete Lesson 20 in the *Virtual Patient Encounters Study Guide* after you have reviewed the topic in class.

## ▪ Topic Review

### *Objectives:*

*On completion of this lesson, the student will be able to perform the following:*
- Describe how the phases of trauma care relate to a particular case.
- Describe how each component of the trauma system can affect this patient's outcome.
- Relate your knowledge of mechanism of injury to predict possible injury patterns in selected cases.

### *Review the following topics with your students before they complete the lesson:*

- Unintentional injury is the leading cause of death in Americans between the ages of 1 and 34 years.
- Prehospital providers play a key role in preventing injuries and mitigating their effects. Interventions occur in the preincident, incident, and postincident phases of trauma.
- Preincident phase activities involve community education. Incident actions are aimed at preventing injuries to the paramedic or others on the scene. Postincident phase activities involve patient care and taking the patient to an appropriate hospital in a timely manner.
- The severity of injury is related to many factors. Chief among these factors is the amount of energy that is applied to the body. As the energy increases, injury increases.
- Paramedics should consider the mechanism of injury, force of energy applied, what anatomic area is involved, and other energy factors, including mass, velocity, distance between the energy source and the patient, and the energy form.

- The severity of injuries related to falls depend on the distance fallen, what body region impacts the landing surface, and the ability of the landing surface to absorb energy.
- Injuries sustained as a result of penetrating trauma depend on two forces: (1) crushing and (2) stretching.
- These forces in penetrating injury relate to the nature of the penetrating object, its speed of penetration, and the type of body tissue through which it passes.

# Follow-Up

### Assignment follow-up from previous class:

- What problems, if any, did you have with your assignment?
- What questions do you have?

### In-class activities and discussion questions:

- Search an online video site using the words crash or fall to find video clips that demonstrate potential for significant mechanism of injury. Show several brief clips of video images from the site, and have students predict injuries based on the kinematics they see. Ask students to explain the forces that will contribute to the injuries and how the body organs will respond to the forces that are transmitted internally.
- Identify some possible preincident phase activities paramedics can do to prevent injuries.

### Summary assessment:

- Administer the quiz related to this lesson (Evolve resources, instructor's test bank).

# STUDY GUIDE ANSWERS

### EXERCISE 1 ■ Case 7: 8-year-old male—submersion

1. Describe the paramedic's role in each phase of trauma care as it relates to this type of injury.

| Phase of Care | Possible Paramedic Actions for this Type of Injury |
|---|---|
| Before incident | Provide education in the schools regarding water safety. |
| Incident | Exercise safety around the water. If the patient had been in the water when you arrived, then enter only after employing appropriate safety measures. |
| After incident | Maintain in-line spinal immobilization, and manage the patient's airway, breathing, and oxygenation. Assess and treat shock if present. Transport to an appropriate facility for care. |

2. Explain how each of the following components of a trauma system has the potential to affect this patient's clinical outcome.

| Component | Possible Effect on this Patient's Outcome |
|---|---|
| Injury prevention | **Probably no effect. If this child had been educated regarding safe diving, then he might not have sustained the injury.** |
| Prehospital care | **Appropriate prehospital care will establish and maintain spinal immobilization and adequate oxygenation and ventilation. Transport to the closest, most appropriate facility.** |
| Emergency department care | **Emergency department care will focus on making arrangements for specialty care to stabilize the spinal injury and on identifying and treating other concurrent injuries.** |
| Interfacility transport | **If transport to a specialty center is not possible from the scene, then interfacility transfer of this patient to a trauma center for definitive care is important to increase the patient's chance for a favorable outcome.** |
| Definitive care | **A specialty center provides definitive care for this patient's condition to stabilize the spine and prevent further injury.** |
| Trauma critical care | **Appropriate critical care is essential to mitigate complications of spinal cord injury. These complications can include blood clots, infections, and skin breakdown, among others. Specialty care can minimize the incidence of these complications.** |
| Rehabilitation | **After the acute phase of care, appropriate rehabilitation will be needed to assist this patient to relearn activities of daily living such as moving about (in a wheelchair), transferring from wheelchair to bed and bathing.** |
| Data collection and trauma registry | **Data collection and trauma registry can identify factors that improve outcomes or target specific regions for selected injury prevention programs.** |

3. This patient was injured in a vertical fall. The three factors that influence injury in this type of fall are (1) the distance fallen, (2) the body position of the patient on impact, and (3) the type of landing surface. Explain the role of each factor in the injuries that this patient sustained.

| Factors that Influence Injury after a Fall | How Do these Factors Influence Injury in this Case? |
|---|---|
| Distance fallen | **Unclear whether patient dove from deck level or from an elevated board or platform.** |
| Body position | **In many instances, the dive injury strikes the forehead and causes hyperextension of the head, forcing the spinal column past its normal range of motion.** |
| Type of landing surface | **Video shows that this child would have struck a very hard surface.** |

### EXERCISE 2 ■ *Case 11: 32-year-old male—gunshot wounds*

4. Describe interventions that may be taken by paramedics to reduce the incidence of death in each period in which trauma deaths occur.

| Periods of Trauma Deaths | Paramedic Interventions to Reduce Incidence of Deaths |
| --- | --- |
| Immediate | **Open the airway, assist ventilations, and cover open wounds on thorax and neck.** |
| Early | **Immobilize spinal column, initiate intravenous therapy, and provide fluid volume replacement while providing rapid transport to a trauma center.** |
| Late | **Take measures to prevent infection, respiratory failure, and renal failure. Use aseptic technique when establishing intravenous access, ensure adequate ventilation and oxygenation, and treat the patient for shock.** |

5. Kinetic energy is equal to one-half the mass multiplied by the velocity squared:

$$KE = (m/2) \times V^2$$

Explain the factors in a shooting that influence tissue damage as they relate to the above formula.

**Kinetic energy and therefore the amount of tissue damage will be related to *mass* and velocity. The tissue damage is not only related to the actual size of the bullet, but it is also related to the part of the bullet that first strikes the tissue—if the point strikes first, then the damage will be less than if the bullet enters the tissue sideways. As the speed of a bullet increases, the amount of cavitation and tissue damage will increase. The distance or range at which the bullet was fired from the patient also influences velocity. Air drag will decrease the bullet velocity if it travels a long distance. Examples of medium-energy weapons are handguns and some rifles. Military assault rifles are high-velocity weapons.**

# Multisystem Trauma

## ■ Assignment

### Prerequisites:

- Complete Chapter 21, Hemorrhage and Shock; Chapter 24, Head and Facial Trauma; Chapter 25, Spinal Trauma; Chapter 26, Thoracic Trauma; and Chapter 27, Abdominal Trauma, in *Mosby's Paramedic Textbook, Revised Third Edition.*
- Complete Chapters 21, 24, 25, 26, and 27 in the workbook for *Mosby's Paramedic Textbook, Revised Third Edition.*
- Complete any skills or laboratory studies pertinent to this lesson.
- Read the "Getting Started" and "Orientation to Virtual Patient Encounters" sections in the *Virtual Patient Encounters Study Guide* (if this is the first lesson being attempted).

### Other relevant chapters:

In addition to Chapters 21, 24, 25, 26, and 27, this lesson also draws content found in the following chapters:

- Chapter 2, The Well-Being of the Paramedic
- Chapter 4, Medical/Legal Issues
- Chapter 6, Review of Human Systems
- Chapter 7, General Principles of Pathophysiology
- Chapter 11, Techniques of Physical Examination
- Chapter 12, Patient Assessment
- Chapter 16, Documentation
- Chapter 18, Venous Access and Medication Administration
- Chapter 19, Airway Management and Ventilation
- Chapter 20, Trauma Systems and Mechanism of Injury
- Chapter 22, Soft Tissue Trauma
- Chapter 52, Crime Scene Awareness

### Student assignment:

- Complete Lesson 21 in the *Virtual Patient Encounters Study Guide* after you have reviewed the topic in class.

# ◼ Topic Review

### Objectives:

*On completion of this lesson, the student will be able to perform the following:*

- Demonstrate appropriate actions to take when responding to a patient injured by gunshots.
- Predict the injuries from penetrating trauma based on the knowledge of anatomy and physiology.
- Manage life threats, including airway, breathing, and circulatory problems, for the patient with penetrating trauma.

### Review the following topics with your students before they complete the lesson:

- Scene safety is always the first consideration when responding to a call involving a gunshot wound. Stage at a safe distance until the dispatcher instructs you to approach the scene. Don appropriate body substance isolation (BSI) gear before you approach the scene. Remain vigilant throughout the call if there is any question about the status of the perpetrator.
- Perform the initial assessment, and address life-threatening conditions as they are found. If a wound is found to the torso or abdomen, then assess for the presence of bilateral breath sounds during the initial assessment.
- Remove or cut clothing quickly so you can identify entry and exit wounds. Once the wounds are identified, you can predict the internal damage based on the trajectory of the wounding missile.
- Wounds to the chest should always be treated as open wounds until proven otherwise. Keep in mind that the top of each lung extends above the clavicle. In addition, wounds of the upper abdomen can easily penetrate the chest cavity, depending on the path of the bullet.
- Be sure to expose and examine the patient's body quickly to ensure that you do not miss any injuries. Check the entire anterior surface, inspect the axilla, and log roll the patient to inspect the patient's back for wounds.
- Patients with penetrating injuries often need surgical intervention. Patient care and transport must be provided quickly to maximize the patient's chances of survival. Ensure adequate airway, breathing, and circulation, and then start intravenous (IV) lines en route to the hospital. Your goal should be to treat and transport within 10 minutes of your arrival on the scene.
- Be sure to transport patients with gunshot wounds to a trauma center if a center is located within your primary transport zone. Survival is shown to be greater if the patient is taken to a trauma center.

# ◼ Follow-Up

### Assignment follow-up from previous class:

- What problems, if any, did you have with your assignment?
- What questions do you have?

### In-class activities and discussion questions:

- What is the importance of predicting the trajectory of the bullet?
- What interventions are essential for this patient to maximize his or her chances of arriving at the hospital with a pulse?
- List your top three priorities as you arrive on the scene to begin caring for a patient who has been shot.

*Other possible postcase activities:*

- Have students give a radio report detailing their care of the patient.
- Ask the class or a student group to evaluate the radio report.

*Summary assessment:*

- Administer the quiz related to this lesson (Evolve resources, instructor's test bank).

# ■ STUDY GUIDE ANSWERS

### EXERCISE 1 ■ *Case 11: 32-year-old male—gunshot wounds*

1. How do you know that the scene is safe and you may approach the patient?

   **Do not approach the scene until dispatch radios to tell you the scene is safe, which is typically after police have arrived and assessed the situation to determine that no imminent threat exists. You should always still remain vigilant.**

2. What immediate life threats did you identify in this patient?

   **Immediate life threats included unresponsive patient, inadequate ventilation and oxygenation, open chest wounds, and uncontrolled bleeding.**

3. What type of dressing would you apply to each wound? Discuss your rationale for the application of each.

| Wound | Dressing | Rationale |
|---|---|---|
| Neck | Occlusive | If the jugular vein is injured, then air can be drawn into the central circulation and cause shock. |
| Chest | Occlusive | Gunshot wounds to the chest are open wounds until proven otherwise. The potential exists for disruption of the mechanics of respiration because, when the pressure drops in the chest, air will be sucked in through the gunshot wound and less air will enter through the upper airway. |
| Abdomen | Dry bulky | Dressing is used to control bleeding; may need to apply pressure if bleeding is brisk. |

4. List three causes of shock that you identified in this patient. What signs, symptoms, or physical findings led you to the clinical impression in each case? How did each type of shock affect preload?

| Type of Shock | Signs, Symptoms, and Findings that Suggest this Type of Shock | Effect on Preload |
| --- | --- | --- |
| Hypovolemic | Mechanism of injury suggests internal bleeding, tachycardia, skin pallor, hypotension secondary to bleeding inside the chest and abdomen. | Decreased preload secondary to decreased blood volume. |
| Cardiogenic | Absent breath sounds on right lung accompanied by signs of shock secondary to tension pneumothorax. | This status causes decreased preload because blood flow through the inferior and superior venae cavae is obstructed. When increased pressure in the affected lung shifts, the mediastinum shifts and kinks the blood vessels. |
| Neurogenic | Flaccid paralysis of extremities; also warm, dry skin below level of injury secondary to spinal cord injury. | This status causes decreased preload related to a decrease in peripheral vascular resistance; it also prevents compensation for the other types of shock. |

5. Explain the rationale for the airway, ventilation, and oxygenation choices you made for this patient.

   **Initially, the patient was unresponsive, with gasping respirations of 8 breaths per minute and abdominal breathing. The airway needed to be opened immediately by manual means (using spinal precautions because of the wound to the neck). Then, an oral airway needed to be inserted. Ventilation with bag-mask and high-flow oxygen was continued until other immediate life threats were managed, and then the patient was intubated.**

6. Based on the location of the gunshot wounds and the patient's signs and symptoms, predict which organs or significant body structures each bullet injured.

   a. Neck:

   **Blood vessels. A vein was likely injured because bleeding was controlled easily when an occlusive dressing was applied. Evidence suggests that this patient has a high spinal cord injury because of the paralysis and impaired ventilation that is present.**

   b. Chest:

   **Breath sounds were absent on the right side, which indicates probable injury to the lung on the right side. Some blood vessels were likely injured. However, whether pericardial tamponade exists is unclear from the information given in the scenario. (No jugular venous distention, muffled heart tones are noted; however, the patient is hypotensive and tachycardic.)**

c. Abdomen:

**The patient was shot in the right upper quadrant of the abdomen; therefore injury to the liver and possibly the small bowel is likely. Other organs may also be injured, depending on the trajectory of the bullet.**

7. List at least three measures you should take to preserve evidence on this call.

**Cut clothes along the seam if possible; definitely avoid cutting through bullet holes if possible. Avoid disturbing evidence found at the scene. Bag any clothing in paper bags or give directly to police. Document disposition of evidence. Document location and size of injuries as exactly as possible.**

8. Complete a patient care report (PCR) for this call. (Use one of the blank PCRs in the back of your study guide or one your instructor has given you.)

**Each PCR will vary according to the treatment the student provided. Use the following guidelines to score the report. Some suggested significant information that should be noted is also included in italic print.**

## PCR Evaluation Guidelines

| Element | Suggested Completion | Maximum Score |
|---|---|---|
| **Chief complaint** | **Documented appropriately and completely** | 1 |
| **Pertinent medical history** | **SAMPLE history and major medical history is documented accurately.** | 1 |
| | **Example:** | |
| | *S—Three gunshot wounds, one to neck, one to chest, one to abdomen* | |
| | *A, M, P, L—Unknown* | |
| | *E—Police department spokesperson says the patient was shot three times at close range during altercation at bar.* | |
| **History of present illness** | **The events leading up to the illness or injury are clearly and concisely described in an appropriate sequence.** | 2 |
| | **Example:** | |
| | *O—Occurred just before EMS call* | |
| | *P—Three gunshot wounds* | |
| | *Q—Life threatening* | |
| | *R—Unknown* | |
| | *S—Life threatening* | |
| | *T—Just before call to EMS* | |

**PCR Evaluation Guidelines**—*Continued*

| Element | Suggested Completion | Maximum Score |
|---|---|---|
| Physical examination | Appropriate physical examination that includes pertinent negatives is documented in a clear, concise manner using appropriate medical terminology.<br><br>Example:<br><br>*Unresponsive patient has gasping respirations at 8 breaths per minute. Abdominal breathing present. Bleeding is controlled with dressing application. Patient opens eyes and tries to moan and verbalize after ventilation. Breath sounds absent on right but present on left. Pupils midsize, equal, and react to light. Gunshot wound on right side of neck. Gunshot wound on right upper chest and right upper quadrant. Abdomen is rigid to palpation. Skin is flushed on upper and lower extremities. Flaccid paralysis of upper and lower extremities. No response to painful stimulus. Log rolled and back examined; no exit wounds observed.* | 2 |
| Sequence and readability | The narrative is written to convey the sequence of the story clearly and includes relevant details. | 1 |
| Vital signs | Initial vital signs and those obtained after each intervention and patient change are documented accurately and completely.<br><br>NOTE: Vital signs documented should match those obtained in student log. Electrocardiographic data should be documented as sinus tachycardia. | |
| Interventions | Complete documentation of interventions that includes sufficient details.<br><br>*Oxygen administration; measures to clear and maintain airway; ventilation techniques; IV therapy includes volume and rate of administration; specific dressings applied; chest decompression, patient positioning, and other relevant interventions initiated. Includes appropriate treatment based on reassessment of the patient (including specifics related to endotracheal intubation) necessary to evaluate each intervention.* | 2 |
| Total score | | 10 |

## EXERCISE 2 ■ *Summary Activity*

Answers will vary for questions 9 through 11.

# Burns

## ◼ Assignment

### Prerequisites:

- Complete Chapter 23, Burns, in *Mosby's Paramedic Textbook, Revised Third Edition.*
- Complete Chapter 23 in the workbook for *Mosby's Paramedic Textbook, Revised Third Edition.*
- Complete any skills or laboratory studies pertinent to this chapter.
- Read the "Getting Started" and "Orientation to Virtual Patient Encounters" sections in the *Virtual Patient Encounters Study Guide* (if this is the first lesson being attempted).

### Student assignment:

- Complete Lesson 22 in the *Virtual Patient Encounters Study Guide* after you have reviewed the topic in class.

## ◼ Topic Review

### Objectives:

*On completion of this lesson, the student will be able to perform the following:*

- Apply knowledge of factors that influence severity of a burn injury to predict the mechanism of injury in this case.
- Classify burn injuries according to depth, extent, and severity.
- Predict signs and symptoms a patient with a burn injury may exhibit, based on the pathophysiologic understanding of burn injury.
- Calculate fluid volume requirements for selected burn injury cases.

### Review the following topics with your students before they complete the lesson:

- Burns are associated with high mortality, long rehabilitation times, disfigurement, and physical disabilities.
- Burn injury has four primary sources: (1) thermal, (2) chemical, (3) electrical, and (4) radiation. Thermal burns are the most common.
- Major burn injury produces both local and systemic responses. With a large burn, shock can develop and result in renal failure or death.
- Other systemic effects of large burn injuries include pulmonary problems, gastrointestinal ileus, loss of musculoskeletal function, altered immunity, neuroendocrine changes, metabolic changes, and emotional responses ranging from pain to severe depression.

- The severity of a burn injury is determined by its size, depth, body region that is affected, mechanism of burn injury, and the preexisting health of the patient.

- Prehospital resuscitation of the burn patient includes stopping the burning process; maintaining airway, breathing, and ventilation; initiating fluid therapy; maintaining body warmth; keeping the burns covered with clean dressings; managing the pain; and transporting to the appropriate facility.

- The patient should be assessed carefully for inhalation injury. Determine if smoke was present and if the patient was burned in an enclosed space. Assess for burns and swelling of the face, singed nasal or facial hair, burns or swelling in the mouth, stridor, or patient complaints of difficulty breathing or swallowing.

- Administer oxygen to the patient, and intervene early if airway obstruction is anticipated. You must recognize that airway problems will increase during transport because swelling will be progressive over the first 18 to 24 hours.

- Initiate vascular access within an unburned area in an upper extremity, if possible. Fluid should be delivered using the consensus burn formula. Fluid requirements in the first 24 hours are 4 ml/kg of lactated Ringer's solution multiplied by the percentage of body surface area burned. One-half of the calculated daily amount is administered in the first 8 hours after the burn injury.

## ■ Follow-Up

### *Assignment follow-up from previous class:*

- What problems, if any, did you have with your assignment?
- What questions do you have?

### *In-class activities and discussion questions:*

- Divide the class into small groups. Give each group a plastic doll with burns colored on it. Give the group less than 5 minutes to calculate the amount of body surface area that is burned. Then, give the groups several intravenous bags with macrodrip and microdrip tubing. Have each group select the proper fluid and calculate the amount of intravenous fluid to be delivered in the first hour. Ask each group to regulate the intravenous flow to the proper drip rate to deliver the required volume of fluid.

- Have a fellow instructor or volunteer coat his or her hand with melted hair removal wax (or melted wax used in a hospital physical therapy department). Tell the class that the patient was burned after dipping his hand in a deep fryer filled with boiling oil. Ask the class to classify the burn, depth, extent, and severity and to determine whether this patient should go to a burn center.

### *Summary assessment:*

- Administer the quiz related to this lesson (Evolve resources, instructor's test bank).

# ■ STUDY GUIDE ANSWERS

### EXERCISE 1 ■ *Case 9: 22-year-old female—assault*

1. This patient says that she had scalding water thrown on her that caused her burns. What water temperature would have caused her burns, based on the analysis of the time needed to cause tissue damage at each temperature?

| Temperature of Water | Time to Cause Burns | Likely to Have Caused Burns in this Patient? |
|---|---|---|
| 44° C (111° F) | 6 hr | No. Patient said hot water was thrown on her, which would create brief exposure. |
| 44°-51° C (111°-124° F) | Rate of skin damage doubles with each degree of temperature rise | No. |
| 70° C (185° F) | Less than 1 sec | Water was likely in this range to cause partial-thickness burns. |

2. Predict whether the severity of burn injury would have been more or less had this patient been 85 years of age. Explain your answer.

   **The depth of injury would likely be increased in an older adult because the skin thins and loses elasticity as a person ages. This phenomenon decreases the amount of exposure time needed to cause a deep burn.**

3. Describe the pathophysiologic mechanisms that create the blisters found in partial thickness burns.

   **Fluid seeps between the dermal and epidermal skin layers and creates the blisters associated with partial-thickness burns.**

4. Does the patient have injuries that meet the criteria for referral to a burn center? Explain your answer.

   **Yes, she has facial burns, and she has other trauma. Both of these criteria require burn center care.**

5. If this patient had burns covering 30% of her body, then a systemic response to the burn injuries would have occurred. Fill in the missing information related to local and systemic responses during each phase after a major burn injury.

| Phase | Pathophysiologic Charateristics | Expected Systemic Signs and Symptoms | Expected Local Signs and Symptoms |
|---|---|---|---|
| Emergent | Increased capillary permeability; vaso-constriction at burn site | — | Pallor in the area of the burn |

| Phase | Pathophysiologic Charateristics | Expected Systemic Signs and Symptoms | Expected Local Signs and Symptoms |
|---|---|---|---|
| Fluid shift | Arteriolar vasodilation and increased capillary permeability | Decreasing systolic blood pressure; increasing diastolic blood pressure | Blisters in partial-thickness burns; localized wound swelling |
| Resolution | Sodium loss; potassium released into intravascular fluid; continuing fluid loss; hemoconcentration. In severe or electric burns, hemolysis | Increasing shock; urine output is red and shows red cells and is decreased; possible cardiac arrhythmias | Significant swelling at the burn area |
| Hyper-metabolic | Balance between intravascular space and interstitial space Cardiac output increases | Tachycardia; blood pressure stabilizes; urine output increases | Swelling begins to decrease |

6. Use the Consensus Burn Formula on page 566 in Chapter 23 of your textbook to calculate the fluid replacement requirements in the first hour after a burn injury for each of the following patient examples. Calculate the drops per minute in each example, based on the intravenous (IV) tubing drop factor.

| Patient Weight | Percent Body Surface Area Burned | | | Total Volume to Infuse in First Hour after Burn | IV Tubing Drop Factor (gtt/ml) | Drops per Minute to Regulate the IV Fluids |
|---|---|---|---|---|---|---|
| | Superficial | Partial Thickness | Full Thickness | | | |
| a. 60 pounds | 0% | 0% | 40% | 273 ml (convert pounds to kilograms, multiply by 4, multiply by percentage of BSA burned [not including superficial], divide by 2 [one half of fluid is given in the first 8 hours], then divide by 8 to calculate the total amount to infuse in the first hour). | 20 | 91 gtt/min |
| b. 90 pounds | 0% | 10% | 40% | 511 ml | 15 | 128 gtt/min |
| c. 150 pounds | 10% | 40% | 30% | 1193 ml | 10 | 199 gtt/min |
| d. 240 pounds | 30% | 20% | 30% | 1363 ml | 10 | 227 gtt/min |

*BSA,* Body surface area; *IV,* intravenous.

7. Explain the pathophysiologic significance of a circumferential full-thickness burn in each of the following body regions.

a. Neck:

**Airway obstruction and interruption of venous and arterial blood flow are possible.**

b. Upper arm:

**Blood flow in the extremity distal to the burns may be severely restricted or stopped completely.**

c. Chest:

**Decreased chest compliance will occur, tidal volume will decrease, and ventilating the patient may not be possible.**

# Cardiology I

## ■ Assignment

### Prerequisites:

- Complete Chapter 29, Cardiology, in *Mosby's Paramedic Textbook, Revised Third Edition*.
- Complete Chapter 29 in the workbook for *Mosby's Paramedic Textbook, Revised Third Edition*.
- Complete any skills or laboratory studies pertinent to this lesson.
- Read the "Getting Started" and "Orientation to Virtual Patient Encounters" sections in the *Virtual Patient Encounters Study Guide* (if this is the first lesson being attempted).

### Other relevant chapters:

In addition to Chapter 29, this lesson also draws content found in the following chapters:

- Chapter 7, General Principles of Pathophysiology
- Chapter 10, History Taking
- Chapter 11, Techniques of Physical Examination
- Chapter 12, Patient Assessment
- Chapter 13, Clinical Decision Making
- Chapter 16, Documentation
- Chapter 17, Pharmacology
- Chapter 18, Venous Access and Medication Administration
- Chapter 19, Airway Management and Ventilation
- Chapter 47, Patients with Special Challenges

### Student assignment:

- Complete Lesson 23 in the *Virtual Patient Encounters Study Guide* after you have reviewed the topic in class.

## ■ Topic Review

### Objectives:

*On completion of this lesson, the student will be able to perform the following:*

- Using an appropriate patient history and physical examination, establish the cause of the patient's illness.
- Deliver appropriate patient care in a sequence to maximize the patient's chance of recovery.

- Administer the appropriate drugs in the correct manner.
- Recognize and respond appropriately to changes in patient condition.
- Identify resources needed to appropriately care for an obese patient.

### Review the following topics with your students before they complete the lesson:

- When a patient who is clearly ill has a complex and confusing history, information must be gathered quickly to ensure that the appropriate treatment decisions can be made.
- The paramedic professional must be prepared to respond immediately if the patient deteriorates suddenly. What steps can you take to prepare for sudden decompensation of this type of patient?
- When a patient's condition changes suddenly, the steps of the initial assessment must begin again.
- Open the airway, look, listen, and feel for breathing; assist ventilation if it is absent or inadequate; assess circulation; assist circulation with fluids, medications, electrical therapy, or cardiopulmonary resuscitation (CPR) if it is needed.
- Always think ahead to anticipate the worst outcome, which will allow you to prepare mentally and, with the appropriate equipment and team, to manage a critically ill patient if necessary.

## ■ Follow-Up

### Assignment follow-up from previous class:

- What problems, if any, did you have with your assignment?
- What questions do you have?

### In-class activities and discussion questions:

- What information did you gather about the patient's condition in the first 10 seconds of contact?
- What immediate challenges to providing patient care did you observe?
- List at least four possible causes of this patient's signs and symptoms that you believe led to the patient's condition based on the initial history and your first impression of the patient?
- How will you distinguish the possible causes of this patient's illness?

### Other possible postcase activities:

- Have students give a radio report detailing their care of this patient.
- Ask the class, or a student group, to evaluate the radio report.

### Summary assessment:

- Administer the quiz related to this lesson (Evolve resources, instructor's test bank).

## ■ STUDY GUIDE ANSWERS

### EXERCISE 1 ■ Case 2: 56-year-old female—fell

1. What was your impression of the patient when you saw the initial interview and images of her?

   **The patient looks very ill. She is pale and diaphoretic, and she has cyanosis of the face. She has a kind of dazed appearance. When she speaks, she has obvious difficulty and pauses every couple of words to catch her breath.**

2. What was the initial electrocardiographic (ECG) rhythm that you observed?

   **The ECG rhythm is atrial fibrillation with a controlled ventricular response and occasional premature ventricular contractions.**

3. Do you think any relationship exists between the medications the patient is taking and the initial ECG rhythm? Explain the rationale for your answer.

   **She may be taking the Lanoxin to control the rate of the atrial fibrillation.**

4. What illnesses or injuries do you need to rule out, based on your initial impression of the patient?

   **Congestive heart failure, myocardial infarction, pneumonia, exacerbation of asthma or chronic obstructive pulmonary disease, pulmonary embolus, and drug toxicity (from the Lanoxin)**

5. Based on the medications the patient is taking, what medical history do you suspect in addition to the congestive heart failure (CHF) and cardiac problems that her husband reports?

| Drug | Class | Prescription Use |
|------|-------|------------------|
| Lanoxin | Cardiac glycoside | Atrial fibrillation, congestive heart failure |
| Bumex, hydrochlorothiazide | Diuretic | Hypertension |
| Serevent, albuterol metered-dose inhaler | Bronchodilator | Asthma, chronic obstructive pulmonary disease, pneumonia |

6. What challenge related to transportation is evident in the initial video images of this patient?

   **This patient, who is almost certainly unable to ambulate, is a candidate for bariatric care. She is lodged in a difficult position to access.**

7. Describe strategies that you might use to manage the challenges that you identified.

   **Call for additional help. Attempt to move the bed out of the way. Use assistive lift devices (e.g., a bariatric tarp) to move the patient, if available. If the patient has any assistive lifting device (e.g., a Hoyer lift) in the home, then attempt to use it.**

**EXERCISE 2** ■ *Case 2: 56-year-old female—fell* (continued)

8. Assume that you obtained a 12-lead ECG before the patient's condition changed and it appears as shown in the study guide.

   a. Describe your interpretation of this ECG.

      **Anteroseptal infarction with lateral extension. ST-segment elevation is noted in anterior leads V1 through V4 and lateral leads V5 and lead I and aVL. Reciprocal changes are noted. ST-segment depression is seen in leads III and aVF.**

b. What actions should you take, based on these findings?

**This ECG would be one piece of evidence to suggest that CHF resulting from myocardial infarction is the cause of this patient's dyspnea. Measures should be taken as soon as possible to treat this condition. Administer aspirin. If her blood pressure remains above 90 mm Hg systolic, then nitroglycerin can be given sublingually up to three times. This measure might be supplemented with furosemide 80 mg (or per protocol); if no improvement is noted, then morphine might be given. Efforts to move the patient to the stretcher should be made as soon as sufficient help and equipment is available. If the patient's condition has not changed, then transport to the closest appropriate facility where interventional cardiology services could be performed.**

9. Compare the following characteristics of monophasic versus biphasic defibrillators:

| | Monophasic Defibrillator | Biphasic Defibrillator |
| --- | --- | --- |
| Energy level used to treat ventricular fibrillation for first defibrillation if manufacturer's recommendations are unknown | **360 J** | **200 J** |
| Second and subsequent defibrillation energy level (if manufacturer's recommendations are unknown) | **360 J** | **200 J or higher** |
| Current is delivered using pads or paddles? | **Either pads or paddles** | **Either pads or paddles** |
| Adjusts current delivered based on chest impedance before shock delivery? | **No** | **Yes** |

10. After you place the endotracheal tube, you observe the following findings. State what these assessment findings indicate and the actions you would take.

| Finding | Indicates | Actions Needed |
| --- | --- | --- |
| a. Esophageal detector device bulb fills in less than 2 seconds | **The tube is probably in the proper location.** | **Continue to monitor tube placement during transport.** |
| b. Breath sounds are audible over the left lung but absent over the right lung. | **Other vital signs need to be checked and verified in several locations. The possibility of pneumothorax should be considered.** | **Ensure that excessive ventilation volume is not being delivered. Monitor for signs of tension pneumothorax. Report findings to receiving hospital.** |

| Finding | Indicates | Actions Needed |
| --- | --- | --- |
| c. Capnography wave-form is observed<br> | The endotracheal tube is no longer in the trachea, the tubing is kinked, or the end-tidal carbon dioxide ($EtCO_2$) detector is detached. | Assess clinical signs of tube placement and hypoxia. If problem cannot be corrected or tube placement immediately verified by another means, then deflate the endotracheal tube cuff, remove the tube, and ventilate using a bag-mask. |
| d. The end-tidal carbon dioxide ($EtCO_2$) detector alternates in color between purple and yellow after the sixth ventilation. | The tube is probably in the trachea. | Continue to monitor the patient for correct endotracheal tube placement. |

11. For each drug you administered in this case, indicate the volume of drug that you administered and at least one desired effect of that drug.

    **NOTE: Answers may vary according to the treatment followed in the case.**

    **EXAMPLE ANSWER:**

| Drug and Dose | Volume Given | Desired Effect |
| --- | --- | --- |
| Epinephrine 1 mg 1:10,000 | 10 ml | Increase the likelihood of successful defibrillation; increases blood flow to vital organs |
| Amiodarone 300 mg | 6 ml (may be diluted in 20-30 ml normal saline) | Antidysrhythmic |

12. Would terminating resuscitation be appropriate in this case?

    **No.**

    If you answered *no*, then describe why this patient would not be an appropriate candidate for this decision.

    **Termination of resuscitation would not be considered in this case because this event was a witnessed cardiac arrest, no apparent do-not-resuscitate order existed, and the patient had a return of spontaneous circulation when the proper treatment was delivered.**

13. Complete a patient care report (PCR) for this call. (Use one of the blank PCRs in the back of your study guide or the one your instructor has given you).

**Each PCR will vary according to the treatment the student provided. Use the following guidelines to score the report. Some suggested significant information that should be noted is also included in italic print.**

## PCR Evaluation Guidelines

| Element | Suggested Completion | Maximum Score |
|---|---|---|
| Chief complaint | Documented appropriately and completely | 1 |
| | **Example:** *Difficulty breathing* | |
| Pertinent medical history | SAMPLE history and major medical history is documented accurately. | 1 |
| | **Example:** *S—Awoke with labored breathing. Collapsed after getting up from bed. Is weak and dizzy. Denies any previous attacks like this.* | |
| | *A—Beestings, yellow flies, pollen* | |
| | *M—Lanoxin, Bumex, hydrochlorothiazide, Serevent, albuterol metered-dose inhaler* | |
| | *P—Cardiac problems and congestive heart failure* | |
| | *L—Ate last night. Has not taken medications today.* | |
| | *E—Awakened by labored breathing. After getting up from bed, she collapsed beside the bed and was unable to get up.* | |
| History of present illness | The events leading up to the illness or injury are clearly and concisely described in an appropriate sequence. | 2 |
| | **Example:** *O—Patient states onset 6 minutes before EMS called. Denies any problems the night before.* | |
| | *P—Denies pain; has only weakness and dizziness* | |
| | *Q—Denies pain* | |
| | *R—Denies any radiation or pain* | |
| | *S—Denies pain. Weakness is generalized.* | |
| | *T—States condition was present when she awoke.* | |

**PCR Evaluation Guidelines**—*Continued*

| Element | Suggested Completion | Maximum Score |
|---|---|---|
| Physical examination | Appropriate physical examination that includes pertinent negatives is documented in a clear, concise manner using appropriate medical terminology.<br><br>**Example:**<br>*Alert and oriented × 3. Sitting beside bed. Pale, diaphoretic. Three- to four-word dyspnea. Respirations are shallow and labored. Breath sounds initially wheezes. Pulse is irregular and weak. ECG atrial fibrillation with a controlled ventricular rate.* | 2 |
| Sequence and readability | The narrative is written to clearly convey the sequence of the story and includes relevant details. | 1 |
| Vital signs | Initial vital signs and those obtained after each intervention and patient change are documented accurately and completely.<br><br>NOTE: Vital signs documented should match those obtained in student log. | 1 |
| Interventions | Documentation of interventions is complete and includes sufficient details.<br><br>*Airway interventions, oxygen administration, drugs with appropriate route, dose, and rate of administration, IV therapy includes volume and rate of administration, defibrillation intervals, type and energy level, CPR and other relevant interventions. Includes appropriate reassessments necessary to evaluate each intervention.* | 2 |
| Total score | | 10 |

## EXERCISE 3 ■ *Summary Activity*

Answers will vary for questions 13 through 16.

# Cardiology II

## ■ Assignment

### Prerequisites:

- Complete Chapter 29, Cardiology, in *Mosby's Paramedic Textbook, Revised Third Edition.*
- Complete Chapter 29 in the workbook for *Mosby's Paramedic Textbook, Revised Third Edition.*
- Complete any skills or laboratory studies pertinent to this chapter.
- Read the "Getting Started" and "Orientation to Virtual Patient Encounters" sections in the *Virtual Patient Encounters Study Guide* (if this is the first lesson being attempted).

### Other relevant chapters:

In addition to Chapter 29, this lesson also draws content found in the following chapters:

- Chapter 7, General Principles of Pathophysiology
- Chapter 11, Techniques of Physical Examination
- Chapter 16, Documentation
- Chapter 17, Pharmacology
- Chapter 19, Airway Management and Ventilation
- Chapter 30, Pulmonary Emergencies

### Student assignment:

- Complete Lesson 24 in the *Virtual Patient Encounters Study Guide* after you have reviewed the topic in class.

## ■ Topic Review

### Objectives:

*On completion of this lesson, the student will be able to perform the following:*

- Distinguish cardiac from noncardiac causes of dyspnea.
- Perform appropriate interventions for the patient with dyspnea, based on appropriate pathophysiologic knowledge.

### Review the following topics with your students before they complete the lesson:

- When a patient with a cardiac history exhibits difficulty breathing, you must quickly determine if the patient's distress is related to a pulmonary or cardiac cause.

**103**

- History that would indicate cardiac problems includes medications related to heart disease, report of cardiomyopathy, congestive heart failure, heart attack, hypertension, heart problems, or diabetes.
- In an elderly patient or a patient with diabetes who is at risk for heart disease, difficulty breathing alone may signal an acute coronary event.
- Left-ventricular heart failure (LVHF) is often caused by myocardial infarction, which leads to congestive heart failure (CHF) or pulmonary edema. Other causes of LVHF are valve problems and hypertension.
- Key signs and symptoms associated with CHF are paroxysmal nocturnal dyspnea, orthopnea, tachycardia, and crackles. Jugular venous distention (JVD) and pedal edema may also be present if the LVHF has caused right-ventricular heart failure.
- If available, obtain a 12-lead electrocardiogram (ECG) to detect acute ischemic coronary changes in these patients. If acute myocardial infarction (AMI) is accompanied by pulmonary edema, then the left ventricle is usually involved.
- Prehospital management of pulmonary edema and AMI are very similar.
- If pulmonary edema is present, then additional prehospital interventions would include furosemide and continuous positive airway pressure (CPAP), if available.

# ▓ Follow-Up

### *Assignment follow-up from previous class:*

- What problems, if any, did you have with your assignment?
- What questions do you have?

### *In-class activities and discussion questions:*

- Discuss the indications for and advantages of performing a 15-lead ECG.
- The American Heart Association cautions about using nitroglycerin if the patient's heart rate is less than 50 or greater than 100 bpm. Discuss the rationale for these warnings and how it will affect your care of patients with chest pain.

### *Other possible postcase activities:*

- Have students give a radio report detailing their care of the patient.
- Ask the class or a student group to evaluate the radio report.

### *Summary assessment:*

- Administer the quiz related to this lesson (Evolve resources, instructor's test bank).

# ■ STUDY GUIDE ANSWERS

### EXERCISE 1 ■ *Case 14: 65-year-old male—difficulty breathing*

1. While watching the video, did you observe anything in the background of the situation? How could your observations influence your call? What actions might you need to take to address this situation?

   **A persistent sound of a dog barking was heard in the background. Before entering a residence with an unrestrained dog, paramedics should ask the owner if the dog is dangerous. Then, if possible, put the dog or have a family member put the dog in another room with the door closed in case it becomes aggressive when it senses that its owner is in trouble.**

2. What was the significance of the patient's home oxygen?

   **Home oxygen indicates that a patient is persistently hypoxic. In many instances, home oxygen is related to significant end-stage lung disease (chronic obstructive pulmonary disease, asbestosis exposure). In this patient, however, the home oxygen may possibly be related to CHF based on his medicines and physical examination.**

3. List the classification and indications for each of the home medicines this patient takes.

   **The patient's medicines suggest he has a history of ischemic heart disease, CHF, and gastroesophageal disease.**

| Medicine | Classification | Indication | Side Effects |
|---|---|---|---|
| Lasix | Loop diuretic | Treats hypertension or CHF | Hypotension, electrolyte imbalance |
| Klor-con | Electrolyte | Replenishes potassium lost from furosemide administration | Hyperkalemia |
| Nitrostat | Vasodilator | Treats anginal chest pain | Hypotension |
| Acetylsalicylic acid | Antiplatelet | Prevents clotting by decreasing platelet aggregation; used to reduce the risk of AMI | Gastrointestinal upset, hemorrhage |
| Prevacid | Proton pump inhibitor | Treats gastroesophageal reflux disease, erosive esophagitis, and duodenal ulcers | Diarrhea, alteration of absorption of pH-dependant drugs from the gastrointestinal track |
| Lisinopril | Angiotensin-converting enzyme inhibitor | Treats hypertension and CHF | Hypotension, angioedema |

4. What is your clinical impression of this patient? Describe the factors that led you to this determination.

**Pulmonary edema, perhaps caused by an acute coronary event. He has a history of CHF that is significant enough to require home oxygen. He has dyspnea, hypoxia, crackles bilaterally, JVD, and pedal edema. He has heavy chest pressure.**

5. Assume that you had the capability to perform a 12-lead electrocardiographic (ECG) examination and you obtained the rhythm shown in the study guide. Describe your interpretation of the rhythm and whether it is consistent with this patient's clinical picture.

**ST-segment elevation is noted in leads aVL, and V1-V5; ST-segment depression in leads II, III, aVF, and V6; and T waves are tall in leads V2 and V3. This ECG data suggest anteroseptal infarction (large anterior AMI). This finding is consistent with his chest pain, and CHF is common in anterior AMI because it affects the left ventricle.**

6. Describe each drug you used to treat this patient and the desired mechanism of action.

| Drug | Rationale |
| --- | --- |
| Aspirin | **Antiplatelet and antiinflammatory. Associated with decreased mortality in AMI. Given because patient is on low-dose aspirin at home and may be taking slow-acting enteric form.** |
| Nitroglycerin | **Vasodilator that reduces preload and afterload would normally be the ideal drug here because it is helpful in the treatment of CHF and AMI; however, it is contraindicated when the heart rate is above 100 bpm, and this patient's heart rate is 120 bpm.** |
| Morphine | **Analgesic and decreased preload and afterload, indicated for both CHF and AMI.** |
| Furosemide | **Loop diuretic that also increases venous capacitance and decreases preload; helpful to treat pulmonary edema.** |

7. List nonpharmacologic interventions for this patient and your rationale for using them.

**Patient position: Initially, have the patient sit upright, with legs dependent to reduce preload. For transport, place the patient in a high Fowler's position or position of comfort. If available, a CPAP mask should be applied to the patient to treat the pulmonary edema. This device increases alveolar airway pressure, reduces the fluid backflow into the lungs, and is associated with favorable outcomes in a significant number of patients with pulmonary edema.**

8.  For each of the physical findings listed in the following table, describe how you would assess it and the pathophysiologic significance of each finding.

| Finding | Assessment Technique | Significance |
| --- | --- | --- |
| Crackles in the lungs | **Place the diaphragm of the stethoscope on the patient's bare chest. Auscultate over the posterior chest, from top to bottom, moving from side to side to compare sounds; then, listen anteriorly in the same manner. Have the patient breathe in and out slowly with the mouth open while you listen to the chest. Crackles are usually heard at the end of inspiration and resemble a fine *popping* sound.** | **Crackles indicate fluid in the lungs, either from CHF or pneumonia. Typically, crackles heard in pneumonia are unilateral (unless bilateral CHF crackles are first heard in the bases) and move higher as the patient's condition worsens.** |
| Jugular venous distention | **Evaluate with the patient's head elevated 45 degrees.** | **JVD indicates an increase in central venous pressure, which is associated with right-ventricular heart failure, the cause of which is often LVHF.** |
| Pedal edema | **Press a finger firmly on the lower leg. When you release, observe for an indentation (a pit) in the skin. The deeper the indention is, the greater the edema will be. A value of +1 is a minor depression that disappears quickly; +4 pitting edema produces obvious gross deformity of the skin that remains for greater than 2 minutes.** | **The edema may be caused by an increase in hydrostatic pressure (secondary to right-ventricular heart failure) or venous insufficiency, a decrease in plasma oncotic pressure (decreased plasma protein), an increase in capillary permeability (sepsis, burns), or lymphatic obstruction (after lymph nodes removed in the groin for lymphoma).** |

9.  Explain how the use of capnography might influence your treatment decisions for this patient.

**Capnography monitoring would provide valuable information related to the ventilation status of the patient. You would look at the waveform to assess for bronchoconstriction, demonstrated by a shark fin–shaped waveform. Additionally, you would monitor the carbon dioxide level to observe for signs of decompensation and respiratory failure, indicated by a tall waveform and carbon dioxide levels exceeding 45 mm Hg.**

10. Complete a patient care report (PCR) for this call. (Use one of the blank PCRs in the back of your study guide or one your instructor has given you).

    **Each patient care report will vary according to the treatment the student provided. Use the following guidelines to score the report. Some suggested significant information that should be noted is also included in italic print.**

### PCR Evaluation Guidelines

| Element | Suggested Completion | Maximum Score |
|---|---|---|
| Chief complaint | Documented appropriately and completely<br><br>**Example:**<br><br>*Difficulty breathing* | 1 |
| Pertinent medical history | SAMPLE history and major medical history is documented accurately.<br><br>**Example:**<br><br>*S—Shortness of breath for 2 days. Nonradiating chest pressure started today. Patient is diaphoretic, nauseated, in tripod position. He has pedal edema and a wet cough.*<br><br>*A—Penicillin*<br><br>*M—Lasix 40 mg, Klor-con, Nitrostat 0.4 mg tabs, ASA 81 mg qd, Prevacid, Lisinopril.*<br><br>*P—Heart disease*<br><br>*L—Toast and coffee 4 hours ago*<br><br>*E—Dyspnea has increased over last 2 days. Cough has kept patient from sleeping. He is orthopneic, feels weak, and is getting tired.* | 1 |
| History of present illness | The events leading up to the illness or injury are clearly and concisely described in an appropriate sequence.<br><br>**Example:**<br><br>*O—As above*<br><br>*P—Dyspnea increases when lying, with exertion, or leaning back.*<br><br>*Q—"Heavy" chest pressure*<br><br>*R—Denies*<br><br>*S—10/10 "worse than ever"*<br><br>*T—Began 2 days ago and is now intolerable.* | 2 |

## PCR Evaluation Guidelines—*Continued*

| Element | Suggested Completion | Maximum Score |
|---|---|---|
| Physical examination | Appropriate physical examination that includes pertinent negatives is documented in a clear, concise manner using appropriate medical terminology.<br><br>**Example:**<br><br>*Alert and oriented* × *3. Rapid, labored respirations. Crackles auscultated bilaterally in lung fields. Heart rate 116 and irregular. Pupils equal and react to light. Jugular venous distention present. Using accessory muscles to breathe. Nail beds are cyanotic. Pedal edema is present.* | 2 |
| Sequence and readability | The narrative is written to clearly convey the sequence of the story and includes relevant details. | 1 |
| Vital signs | Initial vital signs and those obtained after each intervention and patient change are documented accurately and completely.<br><br>**NOTE:** Vital signs documented should match those obtained in student log. ECG data should be documented as sinus tachycardia with unifocal premature ventricular contractions. | 1 |
| Interventions | Complete documentation of interventions that includes sufficient details.<br><br>*Oxygen administration, drugs with appropriate route, dose, and rate of administration, IV therapy includes volume and rate of administration. Patient positioning and other relevant interventions. Includes appropriate reassessments necessary to evaluate each intervention.* | 2 |
| **Total score** | | **10** |

## EXERCISE 2 ■ *Summary Activity*

Answers will vary for questions 11 through 14.

# Pulmonary Emergencies

## ■ Assignment

### Prerequisites:

- Complete Chapter 30, Pulmonary Emergencies, in *Mosby's Paramedic Textbook, Revised Third Edition*.
- Complete Chapter 30 in the workbook for *Mosby's Paramedic Textbook, Revised Third Edition*.
- Complete any skills or laboratory studies pertinent to this chapter.
- Read the "Getting Started" and "Orientation to Virtual Patient Encounters" sections in the *Virtual Patient Encounters Study Guide* (if this is the first lesson being attempted).

### Other relevant chapters:

In addition to Chapter 30, this lesson also draws content found in the following chapters:
- Chapter 2, The Well-Being of the Paramedic
- Chapter 7, General Principles of Pathophysiology
- Chapter 10, History Taking
- Chapter 11, Techniques of Physical Examination
- Chapter 12, Patient Assessment
- Chapter 16, Documentation
- Chapter 17, Pharmacology
- Chapter 18, Venous Access and Medication Administration
- Chapter 39, Infectious and Communicable Diseases

### Student assignment:

- Complete Lesson 25 in the *Virtual Patient Encounters Study Guide* after you have reviewed the topic in class.

## ■ Topic Review

### Objectives:

*On completion of this lesson, the student will be able to perform the following:*
- Form a clinical impression based on a careful history and physical examination.
- Identify key interventions needed to effect a favorable outcome for the patient.
- Recognize the appropriateness of safety interventions for emergency medical services (EMS) personnel in this case.

### *Review the following topics with your students before they complete the lesson:*

- In some cases of difficulty breathing, no abnormal findings will be noted when you listen to lungs with a stethoscope. Without a thorough history and physical examination, the paramedic may misinterpret the nature of illness.

- In cases in which hypoxia and severe dyspnea are evident, misinterpreting the nature of illness is unlikely. However, when symptoms are somewhat vague and vital sign findings are borderline, failure to obtain a thorough history and perform a focused physical examination might lead to disaster.

- Interpreting rapid respirations with tingling around the lips as mere hyperventilation related to an anxiety attack is easy for the inexperienced paramedic.

- Application of a paper bag over the face of a patient with hypoxia can lead to rapid deterioration of the patient.

- When in doubt, err on the side of caution. Expect an underlying pathologic abnormality that you do not have the proper training or equipment to assess properly. In addition, ensure that the patient is transported to the appropriate medical facility.

- If you cannot identify a cause for the dyspnea, treat the patient's symptoms. Administer oxygen, and transport quickly in a position of comfort. Perform a 12-lead electrocardiographic (ECG) assessment, and monitor the three-lead ECG to detect any changes en route.

- The paramedic must continuously monitor the patient's condition in case of changes. Reassess vital signs and oxygen saturation ($SaO_2$) at least every 15 minutes—every 5 minutes if an abnormality is identified.

## ■ Follow-Up

### *Assignment follow-up from previous class:*

- What problems, if any, did you have with your assignment?
- What questions do you have?

### *In-class activities and discussion questions:*

- If you have access to a monitor with waveform capnography, connect yourself or a student to the carbon dioxide ($CO_2$) monitor and the $SaO_2$ monitor. Breathe fast and then slow, and then hold your breath. Have the class compare and contrast the changes in $SaO_2$, end-tidal $CO_2$, and your rate and depth of breathing with each change in ventilation.

- Have the students discuss the mechanism by which pulmonary emboli impair oxygenation.

### *Other possible postcase activities:*

- Have students give a radio report detailing their care of the patient.
- Ask the class or a student group to evaluate the radio report.

### *Summary assessment:*

- Administer the quiz related to this lesson (Evolve resources, instructor's test bank).

# ■ STUDY GUIDE ANSWERS

## EXERCISE 1 ■ *Case 15: 42-year-old male—difficulty breathing*

1. What is your clinical impression of this patient? Describe the historical and physical assessment cues that led you to that impression.

   **Clinical impression is pulmonary embolus.**

   | History | Physical Examination |
   |---|---|
   | Long trip in a motor vehicle with prolonged immobility; recently had cast removed from leg for ankle fracture; aching in his chest for 2 weeks; aching chest pain | Dyspnea, hypoxia, tachycardia, tachypnea, jugular vein distention |

2. What are your highest priorities for care for this patient?

   **The priorities of care are to administer high-concentration oxygen and transport the patient urgently to the closest appropriate facility. If a fibrinolytic inclusion-exclusion criteria form is available in the ambulance, complete it. Tell the physician your suspicion in the radio report so rapid evaluation and treatment can begin in the emergency department.**

3. What electrocardiographic (ECG) rhythm did you observe? What is causing the rhythm? How will you manage it?

   **The ECG showed sinus tachycardia with frequent premature ventricular contractions, which is likely related to his hypoxia. No drugs will be given to control the rhythm unless ordered by a physician.**

4. Explain why you selected the oxygen device and flow rate that you chose.

   **Because the patient is hypoxic (low $SaO_2$, dyspnea, cyanosis), the nonrebreather mask is set at 12 to 15 L/min.**

5. Was it appropriate for the paramedics to apply the masks? Explain your answer.

   **Paramedics should follow local protocols related to personal protective equipment (PPE). If the patient has been taking his tuberculosis medicine, then he is not likely contagious. If, after questioning him and his wife, any indication exists that he is noncompliant with medication, then the appropriate PPE should be worn, especially if he is coughing. In this scenario, the masks the paramedics wear are not N-95 or high-efficiency particulate air filter masks and would not be appropriate if the patient was contagious with tuberculosis.**

6. Describe the pathophysiologic cause of the signs and symptoms you observed in the patient as they relate to your clinical impression.

| Sign or Symptom | Pathophysiologic Cause |
| --- | --- |
| Dyspnea | **If a large clot is present in the pulmonary artery, it will prevent blood from reaching the alveoli to pick up oxygen from the blood. A perfusion-ventilation mismatch will occur. Although enough oxygen is being inhaled and getting to the alveoli, some of the respiratory membrane is not being perfused.** |
| Jugular venous distention (JVD) | **Blood vessels that are blocked with a clot produce vasoconstriction and pulmonary hypertension, a condition that causes blood to back up in the right side of the heart and into the jugular veins.** |
| Decreased SaO$_2$ | **Although oxygen is getting to the alveoli, some of the alveoli have no blood flowing past them to pick up oxygen and deliver it to the cells; thus SaO$_2$ levels drop (depending on size of clot).** |

7. The patient has tingling around his lips. Why do you think this sign is not hyperventilation related to an anxiety attack?

**The hyperventilation this patient has is related to hypoxia, as seen by the low SaO$_2$ and cyanosis. If you were to treat this patient for hyperventilation, you might cause increased hypoxia and death.**

8. Distinguish the assessment findings for each of the following causes of respiratory distress. Then identify whether any of these findings are found in this patient.

| Disease | Breath Sounds | History of Present Illness | Medical History | Home Medicines (if history of the illness is known) |
| --- | --- | --- | --- | --- |
| Pulmonary edema | **Crackles bilaterally** | **Sudden onset, awakened from sleep with dyspnea, orthopnea** | **Hypertension, heart disease, myocardial infarction, congestive heart failure, cardiomyopathy** | **Angiotensin-converting enzyme inhibitors, Coreg, digoxin, spironolactone, Lasix, Bumex, other diuretics** |
| *Found in this patient?* | **No** | **No** | **No** | **No** |
| Anaphylaxis | **Inspiratory and expiratory wheezes, diminished breath sounds throughout** | **History of exposure to known allergen; other findings may include erythema, urticaria, hypotension, angioedema** | **Known allergy** | **Epinephrine auto-injector, antihistamine such as diphenhydramine** |
| *Found in this patient?* | **No** | **No** | **No** | **No** |

| Disease | Breath Sounds | History of Present Illness | Medical History | Home Medicines (if history of the illness is known) |
|---|---|---|---|---|
| Pulmonary embolism | Localized wheezing | Cough, pain, anxiety, syncope, hypotension, diaphoresis, tachypnea, tachycardia, fever, distended neck veins | Sickle cell disease, hypercoagulability disorder, known deep-vein thrombosis or high risk for same (prolonged immobility, long bone fractures, smoking, pregnancy, sepsis, varicose veins, malignancy) | Birth control pills |
| *Found in this patient?* | No | Tachypnea, tachycardia, jugular vein distention | Cast for fracture, long trip in a motor vehicle | No |
| Asthma | Wheezes | Tachycardia, tachypnea | History of asthma or reactive airway disease | Albuterol, Maxair (or other beta-2 agonists), Atrovent, Singulair |
| *Found in this patient?* | No | Yes | No | Albuterol |
| Pneumonia | Localized wheezes or diminished breath sounds | Fever, tachycardia, cough with discolored sputum | Immunosuppression, influenza | Antibiotic |
| *Found in this patient?* | No | Tachycardia | No | No |

9. Complete a patient care report (PCR) for this call. (Use one of the blank PCRs in the back of your study guide or one your instructor has given you.)

   **Each PCR will vary according to the treatment the student provided. Use the following guidelines to score the report. Some suggested significant information that should be noted is also included in italic print.**

## PCR Evaluation Guidelines

| Element | Suggested Completion | Maximum Score |
| --- | --- | --- |
| Chief complaint | Documented appropriately and completely.<br><br>**Example:**<br><br>*Difficulty breathing* | 1 |
| Pertinent medical history | SAMPLE history and major medical history is documented accurately.<br><br>**Example:**<br><br>*S—Sudden onset of difficulty breathing*<br><br>*A—Denies*<br><br>*M—Rifamate, Tenormin, albuterol metered-dose inhaler*<br><br>*P—Tuberculosis (TB) and hypertension. Recent diagnosis of asthma. Recently had lower leg cast removed after fractured ankle*<br><br>*L—Soup and coffee for dinner 2 hours ago.*<br><br>*E—Just returned from road trip that involved 15-hour days in the car. Physician says his TB is not contagious. He takes all medicines as prescribed. Has numbness, tingling around mouth and nose. Says, "I can't catch my breath." Denies previous episodes of shortness of breath but has periodic "aches" in chest for 3 weeks. Denies complications from TB.* | 1 |
| History of present illness | Events leading up to the illness or injury are clearly and concisely described in an appropriate sequence.<br><br>**Example:**<br><br>*O—Symptoms—"Came on while unpacking clothes."*<br><br>*P—Nothing provokes or palliates.*<br><br>*Q—"I can't catch my breath."*<br><br>*R—No radiation but had "aching" in chest shortly after dyspnea started.*<br><br>*S—10/10.*<br><br>*T—Called 9-1-1 5 minutes after symptoms started.* | 2 |

**PCR Evaluation Guidelines**—*Continued*

| Element | Suggested Completion | Maximum Score |
|---|---|---|
| Physical examination | Appropriate physical examination that includes pertinent negatives is documented in a clear, concise manner using appropriate medical terminology.<br><br>**Example:**<br><br>*Alert and oriented* × *3. Rapid, shallow respirations. Breath sounds clear and equal bilaterally. Pulse present, rapid, irregular. Skin pale and cool. Pupils equal and reactive. Neck veins distended.* | 2 |
| Sequence and readability | The narrative is written to clearly convey the sequence of the story and includes relevant details. | 1 |
| Vital signs | Initial vital signs and those obtained after each intervention and patient change are documented accurately and completely.<br><br>NOTE: Vital signs documented should match those obtained in student log. ECG should be documented as sinus tachycardia. | 1 |
| Interventions | Complete documentation of interventions that includes sufficient details.<br><br>*Oxygen administration, drugs with appropriate route, dose, and rate of administration. IV therapy includes volume and rate of administration. Patient positioning and other relevant interventions. Includes appropriate reassessments necessary to evaluate each intervention.* | 2 |
| Total score | | 10 |

## EXERCISE 2 ■ *Summary Activity*

Answers will vary for questions 10 through 13.

# Neurology

## ■ Assignment

### Prerequisites:

- Complete Chapter 31, Neurology, in *Mosby's Paramedic Textbook, Revised Third Edition*.
- Complete Chapter 31 in the workbook for *Mosby's Paramedic Textbook, Revised Third Edition*.
- Complete any skills or laboratory studies pertinent to this chapter.
- Read the "Getting Started" and "Orientation to Virtual Patient Encounters" sections in the *Virtual Patient Encounters Study Guide* (if this is the first lesson being attempted).

### Other relevant chapters:

In addition to Chapter 31, this lesson also draws content found in the following chapters:
- Chapter 2, The Well-Being of the Paramedic
- Chapter 7, General Principles of Pathophysiology
- Chapter 8, Life Span Development
- Chapter 9, Therapeutic Communication
- Chapter 11, Techniques of Physical Examination
- Chapter 17, Pharmacology
- Chapter 19, Airway Management and Ventilation
- Chapter 39, Infectious and Communicable Diseases
- Chapter 44, Pediatrics
- Chapter 46, Abuse and Neglect

### Student assignment:

- Complete Lesson 26 in the *Virtual Patient Encounters Study Guide* after you have reviewed the topic in class.

## ■ Topic Review

### Objectives:

*On completion of this lesson, the student will be able to perform the following:*
- Describe the rationale for specific scene safety considerations on this call.
- Perform appropriate patient assessments in the correct sequence.

- Interpret signs and symptoms based on knowledge of pathophysiology to develop a clinical impression.
- Indicate appropriate patient management strategies.
- Evaluate the effectiveness of patient interventions.
- Document the call appropriately.

### Review the following topics with your students before they complete the lesson:

- Seizures represent diffuse disorganized stimulation of the brain.
- Causes of seizures are diverse. Obtaining an accurate history and performing a thorough physical examination are critical to determine the cause of the seizure activity.
- Seizures may be related to infectious, metabolic, genetic, environmental, structural, traumatic, hypoxic, or idiopathic causes.
- Management of the patient who has seizures should be focused on protecting the patient, maintaining airway, providing ventilation and oxygenation, controlling the seizure activity with drugs, and identifying and treating the cause of the seizures.
- The means and ability to control the airway will depend on the phase of the seizure and the associated muscle movement or rigidity. Position the airway and insert a nasopharyngeal airway, if possible. Position the patient to minimize the risk of aspiration. Suction any debris or secretions that you identify in the patient's oropharynx.
- Administer high-concentration oxygen. The metabolic needs of the body are great because of the muscle activity during a seizure. Additionally, ventilation may be inadequate because of respiratory muscle involvement.
- Establish intravenous (IV) access if possible so that appropriate medication and, if the seizure is prolonged or the underlying condition necessitates, fluid resuscitation can be performed.
- Benzodiazepines are the most frequent type of medications used to manage seizure activity in the emergency setting. If an IV cannot be established, then consider giving the drug by an alternate route.

## ■ Follow-Up

### Assignment follow-up from previous class:

- What problems, if any, did you have with your assignment?
- What questions do you have?

### In-class activities and discussion questions:

- What challenges would you encounter if you were forced to make a rapid retreat on this call because the patient's father came into the room and became physically violent?
- List at least four possible causes of seizures in children.
- What are your priorities in the care of this child?
- What drug group or class is used initially to terminate seizures? Why is this class used?

### Other possible postcase activities:

- Have students give a radio report detailing their care of the patient.
- Ask the class or a student group to evaluate the radio report.

*Summary assessment:*

- Administer the quiz related to this lesson (Evolve resources, instructor's test bank).

# ■ STUDY GUIDE ANSWERS

### EXERCISE 1 ■ *Case 3: 7-year-old female—seizure*

1. What clinical conditions come to mind based on the dispatch information only?

   **A dispatch call for seizures might indicate toxicity from poisons or drugs, head trauma, hypoxia, dysrhythmia, diseases associated with the brain, infectious diseases, epilepsy, fever, electrolyte imbalance, and other conditions.**

2. Would the age of the patient influence your previous answer?

   **Age can influence the possible causes of seizure:**

   **a. Infants—birth trauma, infectious disease, abuse**

   **b. Children—trauma, fever, infectious disease, accidental overdose or poisoning, epilepsy, congenital illness**

   **c. Teens or young adults—trauma, drug overdose, hypoxia from erotic asphyxia**

   **d. Older adults—stroke, trauma, electrolyte abnormalities**

3. What electrocardiographic (ECG) rhythm did you observe? What could be causing this rhythm in this patient?

   **Sinus tachycardia. In this patient, tachycardia might be related to fever, infection, shock, increased metabolism related to muscle activity associated with the seizure, or hypoxia cause by inadequate respirations.**

4. Explain why you performed the airway interventions you selected.

   **An attempt was made to open the airway using manual maneuvers. Insertion of a naso-pharyngeal airway (patient still has a gag reflex) and administration of high-flow oxygen assisted with a bag-mask were performed because breathing is ineffective, as shown by shallow respirations, decreased oxygen saturation, and cyanosis.**

5. Describe the rationale for safety interventions that the crew used on this call.

   **The crew radioed for police back-up when it was evident that the father was displaying aggressive behavior (shouting, slamming doors, saying that emergency medical services [EMS] should not have been called). If the father had approached EMS personnel in an aggressive manner instead of closing door, then the EMS crew should have retreated immediately. The crew was also observed to be wearing gloves and mask for personal protective equipment (PPE). Because the history of physical examination was suggestive of bacterial meningitis, which is spread by respiratory droplets, both of these actions would be appropriate.**

6. What are some possible explanations for the child's father's behavior?

   **The father might be intoxicated, have a behavioral illness, have warrants, or display other criminal behavior that he did not want law enforcement to see; or he may possibly recognize that his child is very ill and may even be going through a phase of the grieving process.**

7. What illness or injury do you believe has caused this child's signs and symptoms?

   **The presenting signs and symptoms suggest sepsis associated with bacterial infection, such as meningococcemia. They include fever, altered consciousness or seizures, signs of shock, and petechiae.**

8. Describe the characteristics of petechiae.

   **Petechiae are lesions that are reddish purple in color. They do not blanch when compressed and are less than 0.5 cm in diameter. When petechial lesions expand beyond this size, the lesions are referred to as purpura.**

9. This child had petechiae on her trunk and extremities. How might your clinical impression have changed if the petechiae were on her head and face only?

   **Petechiae that occur only above the clavicles are typically associated with increased pressure in the upper body. This condition may be associated with abuse, strangulation, or very forceful coughing or vomiting. When the lesions are found below the clavicles in a diffuse pattern, they signal systemic illness.**

10. Describe the characteristics of this child that make her susceptible to abuse.

    **Her history of cerebral palsy and slow development are risk factors that make her susceptible to abuse.**

11. Under what circumstances would it be necessary for you to be placed on postexposure prophylaxis related to this call?

    **Postexposure prophylaxis may be indicated if the child is diagnosed with *Neisseria meningitidis*. If this cause is identified, then the decision to administer antibiotic to the paramedics will be related to the nature and duration of the exposure and the type of PPE that was used on the call. The emergency department or occupational medicine physician should make this decision.**

12. Describe your rationale for selecting the particular fluid administration type and volume for this patient.

    **Normal saline or lactated Ringer's solution should have been administered in 20 ml/kg boluses because the child was exhibiting signs and symptoms of shock (tachycardia and hypotension).**

13. Distinguish the characteristics of petit mal, partial, and grand mal seizures. Discuss whether this child's signs and symptoms fit each category.

| Seizure Type | Specific or Generalized Focus? | Signs and Symptoms | Age Specific? | How Does this Patient Fit Characteristics? |
|---|---|---|---|---|
| Petit mal | Generalized | Brief lapse of consciousness without loss of posture. Lasts less than 15 seconds. May include eye blinking, lip smacking, or isolated muscle contractions. | Often ages 4-12 | Has lip smacking but is unconscious and has prolonged signs and symptoms. |

| Seizure Type | Specific or Generalized Focus? | Signs and Symptoms | Age Specific? | How Does this Patient Fit Characteristics? |
|---|---|---|---|---|
| Partial | Specific focus | Clonic activity limited to one body part; may be tingling or numbness of a body part or abnormal sensory function. | Not age related | Patient has generalized, not focal, signs and symptoms. |
| Grand mal | Generalized | Sudden loss of consciousness and loss of muscle tone. Tonic phase has prolonged extensor or flexor muscle contraction and apnea (for seconds). Clonic phase lasts 1-3 min and has alternating muscle contraction and relaxation, with hyperventilation, salivation, tachycardia. | Not age related | Has prolonged signs and symptoms. |

14. Indicate two alternatives to the drug that you administered to treat this patient's seizures (include the dose and rate of intravenous [IV] administration). Indicate if this drug could be given by another route (if vascular access was not possible).

| Drug | Dose | Rate | Alternate Route? |
|---|---|---|---|
| Diazepam | 1 mg | Slow IV over 2-5 min | Rectal or IO |
| Lorazepam | 0.05-0.1 mg/kg | IV over 2 min | IO, IM, or rectal |
| Midazolam | 0.1-0.15 mg/kg (max dose 5 mg) | Slow IV over 1-2 min | IO, IM, or rectal |

*IM,* Intramuscular; *IO,* intraoral; *IV,* intravenous.

15. Based on your related knowledge of the patient's illness, what should you tell the patient's mother when she asks you if her child is "going to be okay?"

**You should give the mother honest, simple answers without providing false hope. Because you recognize that this illness has a very high mortality rate, you should carefully prepare the mother for the worst. You can tell her that her child's blood pressure is low and her heart rate is high and that you are giving her IV fluids to try to stabilize this situation. You can tell her that you are concerned that the rash may mean she has a very serious illness and that rapid transport to the nearest appropriate hospital is essential. You should not tell her that her child will be okay.**

16. Graph the systolic blood pressure (BP) and heart rate that you obtained in this call (consult your log); then connect the data points so that each vital sign forms a line. You can use blue ink for the systolic BP and red ink for the heart rate.

   - **Each graph will be individual and based on the interventions that the student selected.**

- If the appropriate interventions were selected, then the student should see a trend of increasing BP and decreasing pulse as the oxygen is administered, IV fluids are delivered, and seizures are controlled.
- Failure to recognize and treat the child's shock adequately might cause a variation in the trend. The paramedic must recognize these variations and adapt care accordingly.

17. Referring to your own graph (see page 158 in the Study Guide), answer the following questions:
    a. What trends do you observe?
    b. How did your interventions relate to the trends you observe?
    c. If the trend reversed at any point, how can you explain that variation?

    **Answers will vary to these questions.**

18. Complete a patient care report (PCR) for this call. (Use one of the blank PCRs in the back of your study guide or one your instructor has given you.)

    **Each patient care report will vary according to the treatment the student provided. Use the following guidelines to score the report. Some suggested significant information that should be noted is also included in italic print.**

    ### PCR Evaluation Guidelines

    | Element | Suggested Completion | Maximum Score |
    |---|---|---|
    | Chief complaint | Documented appropriately and completely<br>**Example:**<br>*Seizures* | 1 |
    | Pertinent medical history | SAMPLE history and major medical history is documented accurately.<br>**Example:**<br>*S—Seizures*<br>*A—Penicillin*<br>*M—Mother gave her pediatric Tylenol this morning for the influenza because her child "felt hot."*<br>*P—History of cerebral palsy, developmental delay, frequent ear infections—last episode occurred 1 month ago.*<br>*L—Drank juice 1 hour ago.*<br>*E—Had a bad cold for a week. Hot to touch since yesterday. Listless, anorexic, and wanted to sleep a lot today. Mother found child seizing.* | 1 |
    | History of present illness | Events leading up to the illness or injury are clearly and concisely described in an appropriate sequence.<br>**Example:**<br>*As above, and seizures began approximately 4 minutes before EMS arrival.* | 2 |

## PCR Evaluation Guidelines—*Continued*

| Element | Suggested Completion | Maximum Score |
|---|---|---|
| Physical examination | Appropriate physical examination that includes pertinent negatives is documented in a clear, concise manner using appropriate medical terminology.<br><br>Example:<br><br>*Includes: Unresponsive patient, with unmeasure-able respiratory rate and poor respiratory quality. Pupils are dilated and reactive. Mouth is open with foamy saliva. The tongue is bruised, and her lips are cyanotic. Lip smacking is present. The skin on her head and neck is pale and free of rash. Breath sounds are clear and equal bilateral-ly. Her chest and abdo-men are pale with petechiae. Petechiae are noted in the antecubital spaces bilaterally and on both upper thighs. No petechiae are observed on her back. Seizure activity is noted.* | 2 |
| Sequence and readability | The narrative is written to clearly convey the sequence of the story and includes relevant details. | 1 |
| Vital signs | Initial vital signs and those obtained after each intervention and patient change are documented accurately and completely (includes times).<br><br>NOTE: Vital signs documented should match those obtained in student log. ECG data should be documented as a narrow complex supraventric-ular tachycardia at a rate of 180/min. | 1 |
| Interventions | Complete documentation of interventions that includes sufficient details.<br><br>*Oxygen administration, measures to clear and maintain airway, ventilation techniques, drugs with appropriate route, dose, and rate of admini-stration. IV therapy includes volume and rate of administration, patient positioning, and other relevant interventions. Includes appropriate reassessments necessary to evaluate each intervention.* | 2 |
| Total score | | 10 |

## EXERCISE 2 ■ *Summary Activity*

Answers will vary for questions 19 through 22.

# Endocrinology

## ■ Assignment

### Prerequisites:

- Complete Chapter 32, Endocrinology, in *Mosby's Paramedic Textbook, Revised Third Edition.*
- Complete Chapter 32 in the workbook for *Mosby's Paramedic Textbook, Revised Third Edition.*
- Complete any skills or laboratory studies pertinent to this lesson.
- Read the "Getting Started" and "Orientation to Virtual Patient Encounters" sections in the *Virtual Patient Encounters Study Guide* (if this is the first lesson being attempted).

### Other relevant chapters:

In addition to Chapter 32, this lesson also draws content found in the following chapters:
- Chapter 7, General Principles of Pathophysiology
- Chapter 10, History Taking
- Chapter 11, Techniques of Physical Examination
- Chapter 12, Patient Assessment
- Chapter 17, Pharmacology
- Chapter 31, Neurology
- Chapter 45, Geriatrics

### Student assignment:

- Complete Lesson 27 in the *Virtual Patient Encounters Study Guide* after you have reviewed the topic in class.

## ■ Topic Review

### Objectives:

*On completion of this lesson, the student will be able to perform the following:*
- Distinguish among key signs and symptoms to form a clinical impression of a patient with altered level of consciousness.
- Identify appropriate interventions for the patient with altered level of consciousness.
- Perform assessment and reassessment in the appropriate sequence.
- Document the call appropriately.

***Review the following topics with your students before they complete the lesson:***

- Because the brain is sensitive to small changes in oxygenation, blood flow, and blood glucose, alterations in mental status may be the first indication of a life-threatening illness or injury.
- An altered mental status may be related to metabolic, hypoxic, structural, traumatic, toxic, environmental, vascular, or behavioral causes.
- Determination of the underlying cause of altered mental status is critical so you can perform the proper interventions.
- A detailed history should be obtained and physical examination should be performed to acquire information needed to develop an accurate clinical impression.
- Additional monitoring devices such as blood glucose and oxygen saturation should be assessed to determine if hypoxia or an alteration in blood sugar are causing or contributing to the patient's signs and symptoms.
- Initial interventions should focus on airway, oxygenation, and ventilation. Alterations in these aspects of the patient's physical examination can contribute to or result from the altered mental status.
- Initiate an intravenous (IV) line if the cause of mental status alteration indicates it or if the cause is unknown. An IV will permit medication administration or fluid resuscitation (or both) if indicated.

# Follow-Up

### Assignment follow-up from previous class:

- What problems, if any, did you have with your assignment?
- What questions do you have?

### In-class activities and discussion questions:

- What are some possible causes of these signs and symptoms in a patient of this age?
- What is the importance of knowing all of the medicines that the patient is taking?
- What key findings would you be seeking on your physical examination?
- How would you have determined his medical history if his daughter were not present on the scene of this call?

### Other possible postcase activities:

- Have students give a radio report detailing their care of the patient.
- Ask the class or a student group to evaluate the radio report.

### Summary assessment:

- Administer the quiz related to this lesson (Evolve resources, instructor's test bank).

# ■ STUDY GUIDE ANSWERS

### EXERCISE 1 ■ *Case 4: 64-year-old male—unknown medical*

1. Based on the dispatcher's information, initial scene observations, and the family's observations, state at least five differential diagnoses that you need to rule out. Describe your rationale for each.

| Possible Diagnosis | Rationale |
| --- | --- |
| Stroke | Older patient, risk factor for stroke (diabetic hx), slurred speech. |
| Intoxication | Older patients can suffer from depression and can be alcoholic (slurred speech). |
| Head injury | The patient may have fallen and has sustained a head injury that is causing the slurred speech. |
| Electrolyte abnormality | The patient may have low sodium, calcium or magnesium. |
| Seizure | The patient may have a brain lesion and be postictal. |

2. What additional assessments did you need to perform to rule out stroke?

   **Analyze the patient using the Cincinnati Stroke Scale.**

   **Alternatively, some systems have their paramedics perform the Los Angeles Prehospital Stroke Screen (LAPSS).**

3. Explain how you would perform these assessments on a patient.

   **Cincinnati Stroke Scale: Ask the patient to show his teeth (look for facial asymmetry), raise his arms out in front, and close his eyes (the inability to raise one arm, or one arm drifts down, is abnormal), and ask him to say something such as "It's raining cats and dogs." Slurred speech is an abnormal finding. If any of the three actions is not normal, then stroke is possible.**

   **LAPSS: Positive findings include age over 45, no history of seizures, symptoms for less than 24 hours, patient is not routinely wheelchair bound or bedridden, glucose is between 60 and 400 mg/dl (this patient does not meet this criteria), and obvious asymmetry if the patient smiles or grimaces, grips, or if the arm drift test is positive.**

4. If you think the patient is having a stroke, would you still treat his hypoglycemia in the same manner?

   **Yes. Given that his blood glucose is only 40 mg/dl, he would be treated for stroke. However, extreme care should be used before administration of oral glucose if he is having a stroke because he may not be able to swallow. In addition, medical direction should be contacted before administering glucagon. An intramuscular injection might cause bleeding if fibrinolytic treatment were given to this man.**

5. If you think the patient is having a stroke, what information would be essential for the hospital to know?

   **Attempt to determine the exact time of onset of signs and symptoms so the physician will know if he meets the 180-minute time criteria for fibrinolytic treatment. In addition, if your district carries a fibrinolytic screening tool, then try to complete it before arrival at the hospital. The physician will also need to know the patient's blood pressure.**

6. Would a high index of suspicion for stroke influence your decision regarding where to transport the patient? If you said yes, then explain your answer.

   **If stroke is suspected, then the patient would be taken to a stroke center (if one is available in your transport region).**

7. Respond to the following questions, based on the fact that the patient is taking an oral hypoglycemic agent:

   a. What additional questions should ask the patient?

   **Ask the patient if he has recently been prescribed any new medication or if he has started to take any over-the-counter medication. Some drugs, especially antibiotics, can alter the metabolism of certain oral hypoglycemic agents and cause unpredictable fluctuations in blood glucose.**

   b. Would the care you administer change?

   **Patients who take only oral diabetic medicines and who experience a hypoglycemic episode should be strongly encouraged to be transported to the hospital even if their signs and symptoms resolve after your treatment. Many emergency medical systems have transport of these patients included in their protocol. The risk of having another sudden drop in blood glucose is high in these patients; thus (1) they must be transported for monitoring, and (2) they must be evaluated at the hospital for a possible cause of the episode. These drugs are metabolized in the kidneys; therefore, renal function may need to be assessed as well.**

   c. Would the information given to the patient change if the patient refuses care?

   **If, despite your warnings to a competent patient, a patient continue to refuse any further treatment or refuses transport despite your explanation that he or she is at high risk for another hypoglycemic episode that might lead to unconsciousness or death, try to do the following: (1) Convince the patient to call his or her private physician while you are on the scene; (2) contact medical oversight if you have not already done so; (3) have a family member stay with the patient; (4) instruct the patient to assess blood glucose at more frequent intervals than normal; (5) ensure that the patient eats before you leave the scene; and (6) tell the patient to call 9-1-1 again if symptoms return.**

8. If you elected to administer oral medication to this patient, then describe actions that you should take before giving it to ensure patient safety.

   **Ensure that he has an intact gag reflex. If you are unsure, based on his level of consciousness, give him a sip of water to determine if he can swallow it. If he cannot swallow water, then do not give him anything else by mouth.**

9. Describe the pathophysiologic basis for the signs and symptoms you observed in the patient on this call.

| Sign or Symptom | Pathophysiologic Basis |
| --- | --- |
| Diaphoresis | Signs and symptoms such as skin pallor, tremors, diaphoresis, and tachycardia result from sympathetic stimulation that occurs when the blood glucose drops. The release of epinephrine is a compensatory mechanism that will hasten break down of liver glycogen in an attempt by the body to increase the blood glucose. The sympathetic stimulation produces signs and symptoms similar to those seen in shock. |

| Sign or Symptom | Pathophysiologic Basis |
|---|---|
| Altered mental status | A cellular deficit of glucose inhibits the production of adenosine triphosphate (ATP) at the cellular level. Glucose is involved in the first step of the three-step process of ATP production—it is needed for glycolysis. The products of glycolysis are then essential for the Kreb cycle. Lack of glucose causes chiefly neurologic signs and symptoms because the brain cannot store glucose. |
| Tachycardia | Signs and symptoms such as skin pallor, tremors, diaphoresis, and tachycardia result from sympathetic stimulation that occurs when the blood glucose drops. The release of epinephrine is a compensatory mechanism that will hasten break down of liver glycogen in an attempt by the body to increase the blood glucose. The sympathetic stimulation produces signs and symptoms similar to those seen in shock. |

10. What age-related factors increase this patient's risk for complications related to diabetes?

**Aging adults may have sensory impairment that can cause errors in medication administration. Some elderly patients also have financial limitations that may impede their ability to buy appropriate food. Major organ function also declines, which can alter metabolism of food and drugs.**

11. Complete a patient care report (PCR) for this call. (Use one of the blank PCRs in the back of your study guide or one your instructor has given you.)

**Each PCR will vary according to the treatment the student provided. Use the following guidelines to score the report. Some suggested significant information that should be noted is also included in italic print.**

**PCR Evaluation Guidelines**

| Element | Suggested Completion | Maximum Score |
|---|---|---|
| Chief complaint | Documented appropriately and completely<br>Example:<br> *"Diabetic crisis"* | 1 |
| Pertinent medical history | SAMPLE history and major medical history is documented accurately.<br>Example:<br> *S—Confused, disoriented, slurred speech*<br> *A—Unknown*<br> *M—Insulin*<br> *P—Diabetes*<br> *L—Unknown*<br> *E—Daughter found her father confused. She obtained a blood glucose of 40.* | 1 |

## PCR Evaluation Guidelines—*Continued*

| Element | Suggested Completion | Maximum Score |
|---------|----------------------|---------------|
| History of present illness | Events leading up to the illness or injury are clearly and concisely described in an appropriate sequence.<br><br>**Example:**<br><br>*Same as above and:*<br><br>*O—Unknown, altered loss of consciousness unchanged through interview.* | 2 |
| Physical examination | Appropriate physical examination that includes pertinent negatives is documented in a clear, concise manner using appropriate medical terminology.<br><br>**Example:**<br><br>*Responsive to verbal stimulus and oriented to person and place. Skin is pale. Pupils are mid-size and react to light. Breath sounds are clear and equal to auscultation bilaterally. Rest of physical examination is unremarkable.* | 2 |
| Sequence and readability | The narrative is written to clearly convey the sequence of the story and includes relevant details. | 1 |
| Vital signs | Initial vital signs and those obtained after each intervention and patient change are documented accurately and completely.<br><br>NOTE: Vital signs documented should match those obtained in student log. | 1 |
| Interventions | Complete documentation of interventions that includes sufficient details.<br><br>*Oxygen administration, drugs with appropriate route, dose, and rate of administration. Patient positioning and other relevant interventions. Includes appropriate reassessments necessary to evaluate each intervention.* | 2 |
| **Total score** | | **10** |

## EXERCISE 2 ■ *Summary Activity*

Answers will vary for questions 12 through 15.

# Allergies and Anaphylaxis

## ■ Assignment

### Prerequisites:

- Complete Chapter 33, Allergies and Anaphylaxis, in *Mosby's Paramedic Textbook, Revised Third Edition*.
- Complete Chapter 33 in the workbook for *Mosby's Paramedic Textbook, Revised Third Edition*.
- Complete any skills or laboratory studies pertinent to this lesson.
- Read the "Getting Started" and "Orientation to Virtual Patient Encounters" sections in the *Virtual Patient Encounters Study Guide* (if this is the first lesson being attempted).

### Other relevant chapters:

In addition to Chapter 33, this lesson also draws content found in the following chapters:
- Chapter 7, General Principles of Pathophysiology
- Chapter 10, History Taking
- Chapter 11, Techniques of Physical Examination
- Chapter 12, Patient Assessment
- Chapter 13, Clinical Decision Making
- Chapter 15, Communications
- Chapter 16, Documentation
- Chapter 17, Pharmacology
- Chapter 18, Venous Access and Medication Administration
- Chapter 19, Airway Management and Ventilation
- Chapter 38, Environmental Conditions

### Student assignment:

- Complete Lesson 28 in the *Virtual Patient Encounters Study Guide* after you have reviewed the topic in class.

# ■ Topic Review

### Objectives:

*On completion of this lesson, the student will be able to perform the following:*

- Establish the cause of the patient's difficulty breathing using an appropriate patient history and physical examination.
- Deliver appropriate patient care in a sequence to maximize the patient's chance of recovery.
- Administer the appropriate drugs in the correct manner.
- Document the call appropriately.

### Review the following topics with your students before they complete the lesson:

- Patients exhibit difficulty breathing related to many causes.
- You must perform a targeted history and physical examination to form the correct clinical impression to ensure care for the patient is appropriately administered.
- If you fail to determine the nature of the patient's respiratory distress appropriately, you might deliver inappropriate interventions.
- Factors to consider when you manage these patients include age, home medicines, allergies, pre-existing medical conditions, history of present illness, and presenting signs and symptoms.
- After you determine the cause of illness, you must prioritize care and deliver the proper interventions in the correct sequence.
- Reassess the patient's condition after each intervention to determine if the patient is responding favorably to your care.
- When you deliver medications to a patient with respiratory distress, wait the appropriate interval before administering a second dose, if it is needed.

# ■ Follow-Up

### Assignment follow-up from previous class:

- What problems, if any, did you have with your assignment?
- What questions do you have?

### In-class activities and discussion questions:

- What desirable and undesirable effects should you anticipate from the administration of the epinephrine autoinjector?
- What questions should you ask the patient to predict the severity of his allergic reaction?
- What findings specific to allergic reaction will you anticipate finding during your physical examination?
- How will you know if this patient's condition is improving?

### Other possible postcase activities:

- Have students give a radio report detailing their care of the patient.
- Ask the class or a student group to evaluate the radio report.

### Summary assessment:

- Administer the quiz related to this lesson (Evolve resources, instructor's test bank).

# ■ STUDY GUIDE ANSWERS

### EXERCISE 1 ■ *Case 1: 20-year-old male—difficulty breathing*

1. What information would lead the dispatcher to state that the cause of the breathing problem is related to an allergic reaction?

   **Caller information might be specific and state that the patient is having an allergic reaction; or the caller may state that patient has an allergy to bee stings, stating that he is stung, has difficulty breathing and a skin rash, or is fainting.**

2. During your initial observation of the scene, what do you notice that might create some difficulty if the patient is transported?

   **The patient is located on the third floor. The location appears to be a college campus but does not appear to be a building with an elevator. If the patient is unable to ambulate, then he will have to be moved down three levels of stairs.**

3. Do the signs and symptoms reported by the emergency medical services responders indicate that administration of EpiPen was appropriate? If you said *yes*, then list the specific findings that justify your answer.

   **Yes. History of allergy to bees, patient reports a bee sting, difficulty breathing, audible wheezes, tachycardia, tachypnea, hypotension**

4. How long must you wait before administering a second dose of epinephrine if it is indicated?

   **The time between doses of epinephrine is 15 to 20 minutes unless the patient is critical. In that case, intravenous (IV) epinephrine might be given without waiting this long.**

5. What was the initial electrocardiographic (ECG) rhythm you observed?

   **Sinus tachycardia**

6. Why would the patient have this rhythm?

   **During shock, the body releases epinephrine in an attempt to increase the cardiac output. Epinephrine increases the heart rate by stimulating beta-1 receptors in the heart.**

7. Explain your rationale for selecting the particular oxygen device and flow rate you selected for this patient.

   **The patient had signs of shock and hypoxia; thus high-concentration oxygen administration was indicated.**

8. What additional physical findings for this patient confirm your clinical impression?

   **Additional signs and symptoms that might indicate anaphylaxis include angioedema, dysphagia, stridor, urticaria, and vomiting.**

9. Describe how the chemical mediators released in anaphylaxis caused the signs and symptoms you observed in the patient on this call.

| Chemical Mediator | Pathophysiologic Effect | Associated Sign or Symptom |
|---|---|---|
| Histamine | **Increases permeability of blood vessels**<br>**Dilates blood vessels** | **Swelling at wound**<br>**Shock (low blood pressure, increased heart rate)** |
| Leukotrienes | **Constrict bronchi** | **Wheezing, increased respiratory rate, dyspnea** |

10. Explain why epinephrine, in the appropriate dose and route, will improve this patient's condition.

   **The alpha properties of the epinephrine cause vasoconstriction, which helps stop the tissue swelling and counteracts the patient's shock by increasing preload. The beta effects of the epinephrine cause bronchodilation, thereby improving the patient's respiratory status.**

11. If an excessive dose of epinephrine were to be given, describe the possible effect it might have on this patient.

   **Excessive epinephrine doses can cause tremors, hypertension, vomiting, myocardial ischemia and serious dysrhythmias—especially if given via IV.**

12. If the administration of intravenous (IV) epinephrine was needed in this case, complete the following information related to its administration:

   a. Dose:

   **0.1 mg (1 ml)**

   b. Concentration:

   **1:10,000**

   c. Rate of administration:

   **Over a 5-minute period**

13. If the only drug you administered was albuterol, would it resolve the patient's signs and symptoms? If you said *no*, justify your response.

   **No. Albuterol is primarily a beta-2 selective stimulant; therefore its action is largely confined to dilating bronchioles. Albuterol may relieve some of the patient's wheezing and dyspnea but will do nothing to resolve the hypotension or any airway swelling related to anaphylaxis, if present.**

14. Explain why this patient needs an infusion of IV fluids.

   **During anaphylaxis, the patient develops shock related to two mechanisms. Increased capillary permeability allows fluid to leak from the vascular space into the interstitial space. The blood vessels also dilate and increase the space in the vascular compartment. Both of these mechanisms lead to decreased cardiac output and shock. If the patient does not respond immediately to epinephrine and still has signs of shock, then 1 to 2 L should be given (up to 4 L may be needed in severe cases).**

15. Describe how your approach to care would change if this patient were a 9-year-old, 40 kg child.

    a. Drug doses:

    **Epinephrine 0.01 ml/kg (max 0.3 ml 1:1000) would be given; for this 40 kg child the dose would be 0.3 ml (1:1000).**

    b. IV fluid infusion:

    **Intravenous fluid would be given in 20 ml/kg (800 ml) infusions (over less than 20 minutes). After the infusion, the child would be reevaluated and another given if indicated.**

16. For each drug that you administered in this case, describe at least two side effects that you should anticipate.

| Drug | Dose | Route | Side Effect |
| --- | --- | --- | --- |
| Albuterol | 2.5 mg | Nebulizer | Anxiety, palpitations, tachycardia, dizziness, dysrhythmias |
| Epinephrine | 0.3-0.5 mg IM (0.1 mg if given IV) | IM (SQ) IV | Headache, nausea, restlessness, weakness, dysrhythmias, hypertension, angina, tachycardia |
| Diphenhydramine | 25-50 mg | IM or IV | Drowsiness, altered coordination, hypotension, palpitations, tachycardia or bradycardia, dry mouth |
| Methylprednisolone | 125 mg | IV | Headache, hypertension, sodium and water retention, hypokalemia, alkalosis |

*IM*, Intramuscular; *IV*, intravenous; *SQ*, subcutaneous.

17. Graph the systolic blood pressure (BP) and heart rate that you obtained in this call (consult your log); then connect the data points so that each vital sign forms a line (see example of page 173 of the Study Guide). You can use blue ink for the systolic BP and red ink for the heart rate.

    • **Each graph will be individual and based on the interventions that the student selected.**
    • **If appropriate treatment is rendered, then the trend should be a steady increase in BP while a steady decrease occurs in heart rate.**

18. Referring to your own graph, answer the following questions:

    a. What trends do you observe?
    b. How did your interventions relate to the trends you observe?
    c. If the trend reversed at any point, how can you explain that variation?

    **Answers will vary to these questions.**

19. Complete a patient care report (PCR) for this call. (Use one of the PCRs in the back of your study guide or one your instructor has given you.)

    **Each patient care report will vary according to the treatment the student provided. Use the following guidelines to score the report. Some suggested significant information that should be noted is also included in italic print.**

## PCR Evaluation Guidelines

| Element | Suggested Completion | Maximum Score |
| --- | --- | --- |
| Chief complaint | Documented appropriately and completely<br><br>Example:<br><br>*Difficulty breathing* | 1 |
| Pertinent medical history | SAMPLE history and major medical history is documented accurately.<br><br>Example:<br><br>*S—Difficulty breathing, audible wheezing on approach to the patient, one- to two-word dyspnea.*<br><br>*A—Bee stings, mold, pollen, dust, mushrooms, penicillin.*<br><br>*M—EpiPen, albuterol metered-dose inhaler.*<br><br>*P—Asthma, severe bee sting allergy.*<br><br>*L—Soup at lunch.*<br><br>*E—Was stung by a bee outside his apartment. Ran up the steps and collapsed. EpiPen administered by first responders.* | 1 |
| History of present illness | Events leading up to the illness or injury are clearly and concisely described in an appropriate sequence.<br><br>Example:<br><br>*As above in E and sign and symptoms:*<br><br>*O—Onset 1 minute after sting.*<br><br>*P—Nothing improves or worsens. Patient is upright sitting in chair "gasping for air."*<br><br>*Q—Burning pain with swelling at site of sting.*<br><br>*R—No radiation*<br><br>*S—Pain at sting is a "3"*<br><br>*T—Onset was about 10 minutes before arrival.* | 2 |
| Physical examination | Appropriate physical examination that includes pertinent negatives is documented in a clear, concise manner using appropriate medical terminology.<br><br>Example:<br><br>*Patient is alert and oriented to person, place and time. Respirations are shallow, with audible wheezes. Initial breath sounds—faint wheezes upper lobes, moderate wheezes lower lobes. Skin is pale. Head and neck: Pupils mid size* | 2 |

**PCR Evaluation Guidelines**—*Continued*

| Element | Suggested Completion | Maximum Score |
|---|---|---|
| | *and reactive, skin pale with cyanotic lips, no angioedema or stridor noted. Chest: ECG— sinus tachycardia, normal chest excursion. Extremities: Arms—normal, puncture wound on left calf is swollen, "about the size of a grapefruit."* | |
| Sequence and readability | The narrative is written to clearly convey the sequence of the story and includes relevant details. | 1 |
| | NOTE: The timing of the administration of EpiPen administration by the first responders is particularly important in this case. | |
| Vital signs | Initial vital signs and those obtained after each intervention and patient change are documented accurately and completely. | 1 |
| | NOTE: Vital signs documented should match those obtained in student log. | |
| Interventions | Complete documentation of interventions that includes sufficient details. | 2 |
| | *Oxygen administration, drugs with appropriate route, dose, and rate of administration. Patient positioning and other relevant interventions. Includes appropriate reassessments necessary to evaluate each intervention.* | |
| Total score | | 10 |

## EXERCISE 2 ■ *Summary Activity*

Answers will vary for questions 20 through 23.

# Gastroenterology

## ■ Assignment

### Prerequisites:

- Complete Chapter 34, Gastroenterology, in *Mosby's Paramedic Textbook, Revised Third Edition*.
- Complete Chapter 34 in the workbook for *Mosby's Paramedic Textbook, Revised Third Edition*.
- Complete any skills or laboratory studies pertinent to this lesson.
- Read the "Getting Started" and "Orientation to Virtual Patient Encounters" sections in the *Virtual Patient Encounters Study Guide* (if this is the first lesson being attempted).

### Other relevant chapters:

In addition to Chapter 34, this lesson also draws content found in the following chapters:

- Chapter 2, The Well-Being of the Paramedic
- Chapter 7, General Principles of Pathophysiology
- Chapter 10, History Taking
- Chapter 13, Clinical Decision Making
- Chapter 19, Airway Management and Ventilation
- Chapter 36, Toxicology

### Student assignment:

- Complete Lesson 29 in the *Virtual Patient Encounters Study Guide* after you have reviewed the topic in class.

## ■ Topic Review

### Objectives:

*On completion of this lesson, the student will be able to perform the following:*

- Perform an appropriate patient history and physical examination to establish clinical priorities of care.
- Establish a list of differential diagnoses based on the clinical findings present in this case.
- Deliver appropriate patient care in a sequence to maximize the patient's chance of recovery.
- Identify appropriate interventions for the patient who is vomiting blood.
- Anticipate appropriate personal protective equipment (PPE) that would be needed on a call with a patient who is vomiting blood.
- Document the call appropriately.

*Review the following topics with your students before they complete the lesson:*

- When you are called to evaluate a patient who is vomiting blood, you must first establish scene safety and then determine whether a traumatic injury is present.
- If you are given "vomiting blood" as dispatch information, you should be prepared and be wearing appropriate PPE when you arrive at the patient's side. These few extra steps can reduce your risk of exposure.
- Your initial impression of these patients is critical. Does the patient appear sick or not sick? Is the airway patent? What is the color of the blood? How much blood does there appear to be?
- Is the patient sick or not sick? Apparent signs of shock can be the first indication that the patient has sustained significant vascular blood loss. If the patient appears ill to an extent that is out of proportion to the amount of blood you see, then more blood may yet come, or the patient may have vomited elsewhere.
- Is the airway patent? Early evaluation and management of the airway is critical. If the airway is patent on arrival, then position the patient appropriately, and prepare to suction in case it is urgently needed.
- What is the color of the blood? The color of the blood can provide clues about the location and nature of the bleeding. Include the description of the blood in the radio report to the hospital so that hospital personnel will know what to anticipate.
- How much blood does there appear to be? The exact amount of blood is difficult to evaluate and is often overestimated. If the patient has vomited into a container, then try to determine an objective measure of the volume.
- Other critical interventions for these patients include general management of hypovolemic shock. If time is available, then establish two large-bore intravenous (IV) lines, which will allow rapid administration of blood on arrival to the emergency department if it is needed.

# ■ Follow-Up

### Assignment follow-up from previous class:

- What problems, if any, did you have with your assignment?
- What questions do you have?

### In-class activities and discussion questions:

- Have students give a radio report detailing their care of the patient.
- Ask the class or a student group to evaluate the radio report.

### Summary assessment:

- Administer the quiz related to this lesson (Evolve resources, instructor's test bank).

# ■ STUDY GUIDE ANSWERS

### EXERCISE 1 ■ *Case 5: 40-year-old male—vomiting blood*

1. Explain why you selected the particular oxygen device and flow rate.

   **The patient was not oxygenating properly, as evidenced by an oxygen saturation of 88%. In addition, with heavy bleeding and signs of shock (increased heart rate and respiratory rate and pale skin), high-flow oxygen administration is indicated.**

2. What safety measures should you and your partner take based on your initial impression of the patient?

   **With the obvious evidence of blood and history of vomiting blood, full PPE precautions should be taken; gloves, gown, eye protection, and mask would be indicated. This precaution would greatly reduce the chance of a significant exposure to blood or bloody body fluids.**

3. What airway equipment should you have ready after you perform your initial assessment?

   **Suction should be ready to use immediately if needed with his history of vomiting blood. Prepare to perform intubation to protect the patient's airway if he loses consciousness.**

4. In what position would you transport this patient? Explain your rationale.

   **Because the patient has signs of shock, you should not place him in a sitting position. However, if you lay him supine, the risk that he would vomit and aspirate increases. Place him in the lateral recumbent position.**

5. List the differential diagnosis (or diagnoses) you should consider in this case based on the following clinical findings. You may select more than one.

   | Findings | Clinical Impression |
   | --- | --- |
   | Abdominal pain | **Cancer, gastritis, gastroenteritis, pancreatitis** |
   | Vomiting bright-red blood | **Esophageal varices, Mallory Weiss tear, perforated ulcer** |
   | Antibiotic therapy for 10 days | **Gastritis, medication reaction, infectious problem** |
   | History of gastroenteritis | **Gastroenteritis, perforated ulcer, esophageal varices, effects of medicines (ibuprofen, aspirin, others)** |
   | Vomits often | **Mallory-Weiss syndrome, pancreatitis** |
   | Pain is associated with drinking | **Pancreatitis, gastritis, peptic ulcer disease, esophagitis** |
   | Pain is intense, nonradiating | **Peptic ulcer, pancreatitis** |

6. What information related to the case might lead you to believe that this patient is alcoholic?

   **The patient gives a history that suggests gastritis or pancreatitis. This illness can be related to alcoholism. He relates that his pain is known to increase with drinking, yet he was drinking at the onset of this episode. The history states that he was "drinking heavily," and that he was drinking liquor and beer.**

7. How does chronic drinking increase a person's risk for gastrointestinal bleeding?

**Alcoholism can lead to cirrhosis of the liver. This damage to the liver destroys liver cells over time and can lead to portal hypertension, which causes a back up of blood in the portal circulation and can lead to bleeding esophageal or gastric varices. The chronic irritation of gastric mucosa from the alcohol can also lead to gastritis. Frequent forceful vomiting can cause Mallory-Weiss syndrome and bright-red gastrointestinal bleeding.**

8. If you measured the patient's blood glucose at 40 mg/dl, you would administer dextrose 50% in water ($D_{50}W$). Based on this patient's history, what drug should be given with the dextrose (include dose and route)?

**Thiamine 100 mg slow IV should be given.**

9. Explain why this is needed and the possible consequences should you not administer it.

**To prevent Wernicke encephalopathy after administration of $D_{50}W$. The body needs the thiamine to metabolize sugar. If thiamine is not given, then the patient may develop ataxia, nystagmus, speech disturbance, neuropathy, or decreased level of consciousness.**

10. Identify the advantages and disadvantages of these fluids as they relate to resuscitating this patient.

| Fluid | Advantages for Use in this Case | Disadvantages for Use in this Case |
|---|---|---|
| 0.9% Normal saline | **Isotonic solution—rapidly expands intravascular volume.** **Crystalloids are cheap and have a long shelf life; therefore they are easy to carry in an ambulance.** | **Two thirds of the normal saline leaves the vascular space within 1 hour; thus it must be given in 3:1 ratio related to blood loss. Crystalloid solutions do not carry oxygen or contain clotting factors. Hypothermia is possible when large volumes of crystalloid fluids are infused rapidly without a fluid warmer.** |
| 0.45% Normal saline | **No advantage** | **This solution is hypotonic and will leave the vascular space quickly.** |
| Whole blood | **Can replace vascular volume and replenish red blood cells to restore oxygen-carrying capacity of blood in the intravascular space.** | **Must be type specific. Requires precise storage temperature conditions. Is extremely expensive. Not practical to carry in almost all ambulances.** |
| Blood plasma | **Can replace fluid volume and clotting factors. ABO compatibility is not an issue.** | **Does not replace red blood cells. Storage considerations and expense make it impractical for prehospital use.** |

11. List at least two disadvantages of large-volume crystalloid fluid resuscitation.

    **Crystalloid solutions do not contain hemoglobin, protein, or blood-clotting factors. When large volumes are given to replace blood loss, the patient's oxygen-carrying capacity will decline, blood clotting will be prolonged, and fluid may leak into interstitial spaces.**

12. Explain whether dopamine would be the first choice to restore cardiac output in this patient.

    **Cardiac output is equal to stroke volume multiplied by the heart rate. Dopamine increases the heart rate and contractility by beta-1 adrenergic receptor stimulation. This action is helpful when managing cardiogenic shock; however, it will not help as a first-line treatment for hypovolemic shock because stroke volume and therefore cardiac output will not improve until intravascular fluid volume is restored. Dopamine should only be used in hypovolemic shock after fluid volume has been replaced.**

13. Why would a patient with a history of chronic alcoholism be less able to compensate if bleeding and shock develop?

    **The alcoholic is often chronically dehydrated, which can result in rapid decompensation in shock. These patients may also have impaired clotting factors, which will retard the normal coagulation process and allow bleeding to continue. If cardiomyopathy related to chronic alcoholic abuse is present, the patient's heart will have decreased contractility, which impairs the ability to respond to shock.**

14. Complete a patient care report (PCR) for this call. (Use one of the blank PCRs in the back of your study guide or one your instructor has given you.)

    **Each PCR will vary according to the treatment the student provided. Use the following guidelines to score the report. Some suggested significant information that should be noted is also included in italic print.**

    **PCR Evaluation Guidelines**

| Element | Suggested Completion | Maximum Score |
|---|---|---|
| Chief complaint | Documented appropriately and completely<br>Example:<br>*Abdominal pain* | 1 |
| Pertinent medical history | SAMPLE history and major medical history is documented accurately.<br>Example:<br>*S—Vomiting bright-red blood. Found with blood over his upper body and on the ground below him.*<br>*A—Denies.*<br>*M—Took an antibiotic for 10 days—ended regimen yesterday.*<br>*L—Was drinking liquor and beer approximately 30 minutes ago.*<br>*E—Drinking heavily, then left bar after onset of abdominal pain.* | 1 |

## PCR Evaluation Guidelines—*Continued*

| Element | Suggested Completion | Maximum Score |
|---|---|---|
| History of present illness | Events leading up to the illness or injury are clearly and concisely described in an appropriate sequence.<br><br>**Example:**<br><br>*Same as above and:*<br><br>*O—States vomiting began approximately 30 minutes before EMS arrival.*<br><br>*P—He vomits frequently and sporadically. Patient states, "It seems to occur mostly after I've had a couple of beers. Then I usually get this awful pain in my gut."*<br><br>*Q—Pain is intense; at times it is 10/10; otherwise, approximately 2/10.*<br><br>*T—Within the last 30 minutes.* | 2 |
| Physical examination | Appropriate physical examination that includes pertinent negatives is documented in a clear, concise manner using appropriate medical terminology.<br><br>**Example:**<br><br>*Patient responds to verbal stimulus and is oriented × 3. Respirations are rapid and shallow. Breath sounds are clear and equal bilaterally. Heart rate is rapid, weak, and regular. Skin is pale, cool, and diaphoretic. Airway is open and clear, with blood splatters on face and neck. Pupils are midsize and react to light.* | 2 |
| Sequence and readability | The narrative is written to clearly convey the sequence of the story and includes relevant details. | 1 |
| Vital signs | Initial vital signs and those obtained after each intervention and patient change are documented accurately and completely.<br><br>NOTE: Vital signs documented should match those obtained in student log. | 1 |

**PCR Evaluation Guidelines**—*Continued*

| Element | Suggested Completion | Maximum Score |
|---|---|---|
| Interventions | Complete documentation of interventions that includes sufficient details.<br><br>*Airway interventions, oxygen administration, drugs with appropriate route, dose, and rate of administration. IV therapy includes volume and rate of administration. Patient positioning and other relevant interventions. Includes appropriate reassessments necessary to evaluate each intervention.* | 2 |
| Total score | | 10 |

## EXERCISE 2 ■ *Summary Activity*

Answers will vary for questions 15 through 18.

# Urology

## ■ Assignment

### Prerequisites:

- Complete Chapter 35, Urology, in *Mosby's Paramedic Textbook, Revised Third Edition.*
- Complete Chapter 35 in the workbook for *Mosby's Paramedic Textbook, Revised Third Edition.*
- Complete any skills or laboratory studies pertinent to this lesson.
- Read the "Getting Started" and "Orientation to Virtual Patient Encounters" sections in the *Virtual Patient Encounters Study Guide* (if this is the first lesson being attempted).

### Student assignment:

- Complete Lesson 30 in the *Virtual Patient Encounters Study Guide* after you have reviewed the topic in class.

## ■ Topic Review

### Objectives:

*On completion of this lesson, the student will be able to perform the following:*

- Anticipate complications of renal failure that can affect patient care.
- Describe appropriate assessment and management of the patient with renal failure.

### Review the following topics with your students before they complete the lesson:

- Chronic renal failure develops over months to years. It can be caused by infection, diabetes, hypertension, or autoimmune disorders.
- Chronic renal failure causes a buildup of fluids and wastes in the blood, including nitrogen and uric acid.
- Complications of renal failure can include hypertension, edema, congestive heart failure, electrolyte imbalances, and anemia, among other problems.
- Renal dialysis is used to treat renal failure. During dialysis, the patient's blood comes in contact with a semipermeable membrane, across which fluid and wastes including nitrogen, uric acid, and electrolytes diffuse into a dialyzing fluid.
- During hemodialysis, blood is pumped through an arteriovenous fistula into a dialysis machine. The fistula connects an artery and vein.

- Peritoneal dialysis involves infusion of the dialysate through a catheter into the peritoneum. The fluid remains in the peritoneal space for several hours, during which wastes and electrolytes diffuse across the peritoneum into the fluid. The waste fluid is then drained.

- Emergencies that can occur during or as a result of dialysis include disequilibrium syndrome, hemorrhage, hypotension, chest pain, air embolism, and hyperkalemia.

- Management of the patient with an emergency related to dialysis will include airway and ventilation support, vascular access, electrocardiographic (ECG) monitoring, and rapid transport. If a treatable underlying cause is identified (e.g., hyperkalemia), then specific interventions should be performed.

## Follow-Up

### Assignment follow-up from previous class:

- What problems, if any, did you have with your assignment?
- What questions do you have?

### In-class activities and discussion questions:

- What if you picked up this patient immediately after dialysis and he began to have seizures? What would you suspect, and what actions would you take?
- If the nurse tells you that the patient has had an air embolism during dialysis, what signs and symptoms would you anticipate? What treatment would be indicated?

### Summary assessment:

- Administer the quiz related to this lesson (Evolve resources, instructor's test bank).

## STUDY GUIDE ANSWERS

### EXERCISE 1 ■ Case 14: 65-year-old male—difficulty breathing

Assume that, in this case, the patient tells you that he was recently diagnosed with renal failure. He has a shunt in his right forearm and had a trial of dialysis 2 weeks earlier, but he missed this week's appointment.

1. How does this information affect your clinical impression of the patient?

   **This information would lead to a strong suspicion that the patient is at risk for congestive heart failure and electrolyte imbalance.**

2. Describe any modification in patient assessment that you must take when caring for this patient.

   **The blood pressure must not be assessed in the arm with the shunt.**

3. How does renal failure affect the oxygen-carrying capacity of the blood?

   **The oxygen-carrying capacity of the blood decreases because the number of red blood cells decreases.**

4. Assume that your patient has the electrocardiographic (ECG) rhythm shown in the Study Guide on page 187. His blood pressure is 70/50 mm Hg, and he has crackles throughout his lungs.

a. In what position will you transport the patient? Explain your answer.

**You will transport him in the position of comfort. He will likely need (want) to sit up so he can breathe.**

b. Interpret the ECG.

**No P waves (disappear when potassium is 7.0-9.0 mEq/L), wide QRS complex (widens when potassium is 6.0-6.5 mEq/L), and T waves are tall and peaked (occurs when potassium is 5.5-6.5 mEq/L)**

5. What variations in the following laboratory values should you anticipate?

| Laboratory Values | Anticipated Variations |
| --- | --- |
| pH | Decreased |
| Potassium | Increased |
| Lactic acid | Increased |
| Blood urea nitrogen (BUN) | Increased |
| Creatinine | Increased |

6. The patient tells you his physician called yesterday and said that he had a high level of potassium. He immediately went into cardiac arrest. You note asystole on the monitor. List the sequence of drugs you will administer to this patient. Explain your rationale for each drug.

| Drug | Rationale |
| --- | --- |
| Epinephrine | Used to cause vasoconstriction |
| Calcium chloride | Used to treat hyperkalemia |
| Sodium bicarbonate | Used to treat metabolic acidosis, hyperkalemia |
| If available, insulin followed by 50% dextrose in water | To move potassium into the cells |

# Toxicology

## ◼ Assignment

### *Prerequisites:*

- Complete Chapter 36, Toxicology, in *Mosby's Paramedic Textbook, Revised Third Edition.*
- Complete Chapter 36 in the workbook for *Mosby's Paramedic Textbook, Revised Third Edition.*
- Complete any skills or laboratory studies pertinent to this lesson.
- Read the "Getting Started" and "Orientation to Virtual Patient Encounters" sections in the *Virtual Patient Encounters Study Guide* (if this is the first lesson being attempted).

### *Other relevant chapters:*

In addition to Chapter 36, this lesson also draws content found in the following chapters:
- Chapter 7, General Principles of Pathophysiology
- Chapter 10, History Taking
- Chapter 11, Techniques of Physical Examination
- Chapter 12, Patient Assessment
- Chapter 17, Pharmacology
- Chapter 19, Airway Management and Ventilation
- Chapter 29, Cardiology
- Chapter 31, Neurology
- Chapter 40, Behavioral and Psychiatric Disorders

### *Student assignment:*

- Complete Lesson 31 in the *Virtual Patient Encounters Study Guide* after you have reviewed the topic in class.

## ◼ Topic Review

### *Objectives:*

*On completion of this lesson, the student will be able to perform the following:*
- Identify priorities of care in an unresponsive patient based on a thorough patient assessment.
- Interpret signs and symptoms based on knowledge of pathophysiology to develop a clinical impression.
- Indicate appropriate patient management strategies.
- Evaluate the effectiveness of patient interventions.
- Document the call appropriately.

*Review the following topics with your students before they complete the lesson:*

- When a patient is presumed to be unconscious, the paramedic should immediately attempt to determine the level of consciousness.
- Initially, the AVPU method can be used, and then a score using the Glasgow coma scale should be assigned to the patient to provide an objective measure of consciousness.
- AVPU signifies that the patient is <u>A</u>lert, responds to <u>V</u>erbal expressions, responds to <u>P</u>ain, or is <u>U</u>nresponsive.
- Glasgow Coma Scale measures best eye opening and best verbal and motor responses.
- Best eye opening is scored from 1 to 4: 4—spontaneously opens eyes; 3—opens eyes on command; 2—opens eyes to pain; and 1—eyes do not open.
- Best verbal response is scored from 1 to 5: 5—oriented; 4—confused; 3—inappropriate response; 2—unintelligible noises; and 1—no verbal response.
- Best motor response is scored from 1 to 6: 6—follows commands; 5—localizes pain; 4—withdraws from pain; 3—flexes to pain; 2—extends to pain; and 1—no motor response occurs.
- After the level of consciousness is determined, the airway should be the priority in the unresponsive patient. The deeper the level of unconsciousness is, the greater is the likelihood that the patient will be unable to maintain his or her airway. Assess and intervene as needed.
- Depending on the cause of unconsciousness, breathing and oxygenation can also be abnormal in the unconscious patient. Evaluate oxygenation and ventilation early in the care, and prepare to perform appropriate interventions.
- Determine the cause of unconsciousness to ensure that appropriate definitive care can be delivered.

# ■ Follow-Up

### *Assignment follow-up from previous class:*

- What problems, if any, did you have with your assignment?
- What questions do you have?

### *In-class activities and discussion questions:*

- What risk factors does this patient have for suicidal behavior?
- If she has taken an overdose of Elavil, then what progression of signs and symptoms should you expect?
- What are your priorities in the care of this patient?
- How might her other disease processes contribute to her presenting signs and symptoms?

### *Other possible postcase activities:*

- Have students give a radio report detailing their care of the patient.
- Ask the class or a student group to evaluate the radio report.
- Review the case again with the whole class, and discuss possible alternative diagnosis or management strategies.

### *Summary assessment:*

- Administer the quiz related to this lesson (Evolve resources, instructor's test bank).

# ■ STUDY GUIDE ANSWERS

### EXERCISE 1 ■ *Case 6: 16-year-old female—unknown medical*

1. What electrocardiographic (ECG) rhythm did you observe?

   **Wide-complex supraventricular tachycardia**

2. Why is this rhythm a significant finding in this patient?

   **Tachycardia with a QRS duration of greater than 0.10 second indicates tricyclic antide-pressant toxicity.**

3. Predict how the ECG rhythm might change if the patient is not treated appropriately.

   **The rhythm could deteriorate into a bradycardia with atrioventricular block, ventricular dysrhythmias, or pulseless electrical activity.**

4. Explain your choice of airway-ventilation-oxygenation device.

   **Her minute volume was likely not adequate because her respiration rate was 10 breaths per minute and chest rise was shallow. Her oxygen saturation was only 88%, and she had vomited and possibly aspirated; therefore, her airway needed to be opened by manual means, an airway device needed to be inserted, and she needed to be oxygenated and manually ventilated.**

5. Given the same initial vital signs (except respiratory rate) observed in this case, select the appropriate airway-oxygenation-ventilation delivery method based on the following capnographic findings. Explain why you chose this device.

| Capnography Reading (Waveform) | Appropriate Oxygen Delivery Device | Rationale |
|---|---|---|
| | Nonrebreather mask 15 L/min | If her saturation level is normal, then you can administer oxygen; she will not require ventilation. The patient may need to be intubated to protect her airway if her level of consciousness does not improve. |
| | Bag-mask ventilation with supplemental oxygen | This waveform indicates inadequate ventilation. Observe her chest rise and fall and respiration rate and pattern. With this type of tracing, she would have irregular apneustic breathing. She would need to have her airway opened and have ventilation assisted immediately with a bag-mask before intubation. |

6. If the patient is anorexic, what electrolyte abnormalities might she have? Could any of these explain the signs and symptoms she is experiencing? Explain your rationale.

   **Patients with anorexia can have a variety of electrolyte imbalances that may include abnormal sodium, potassium, calcium, magnesium and others. Electrolyte imbalances can cause altered level of consciousness, weakness, tachycardia, dysrhythmias, and seizures.**

7. List the drug class and indications for the use of Elavil.

   **Elavil is a tricyclic antidepressant drug and is indicated to treat depression, sleep disorders, and addiction disorders and to prevent migraine headaches.**

8. Explain why ingestion of an excessive amount of Elavil could cause the signs and symptoms you observed in the patient on this call.

| Sign or Symptom | Explanation |
|---|---|
| Altered level of consciousness | **Fast sodium channels in the brain are inhibited** |
| Fast heart rate | **Anticholinergic effects** |
| Hypotension | **Sodium channel blockade in the heart; uptake of norepinephrine blocked** |

9. Describe three other mechanisms that might cause altered level of consciousness or unconsciousness in a patient who has taken an overdose.

   **(1) Some drugs (e.g., narcotics) suppress ventilation when excessive doses are taken. This action impairs oxygenation and can cause altered consciousness or unconsciousness related to cerebral hypoxia.**

   **(2) Cardiac drug toxicity (e.g., beta-blockers, calcium-channel blockers) can cause arrhythmias, profound hypotension, or both. This causes cerebral hypoperfusion and alters consciousness.**

   **(3) An overdose of some drugs (e.g., beta-blockers) can lead to altered consciousness related to hypoglycemia in some patients.**

10. For each drug that you administered in this case, list the class and describe the specific desired effect for this patient.

    **Some drugs that may have appropriately been administered in this case were:**

| Drug | Class | Desired Effect |
|---|---|---|
| **Sodium bicarbonate** | **Alkalinizing agent** | **May reverse cardiac toxicity** |
| **Diazepam** | **Benzodiazepine** | **To manage seizures** |
| **Lorazepam** | **Benzodiazepine** | **Alternate to manage seizures** |
| **Midazolam** | **Benzodiazepine** | **Alternate to manage seizures** |

11. Graph the systolic blood pressure (BP) and heart rate that you obtained in this call (consult your log); then connect the data points so that each vital sign forms a line (see example on page 194 in the Study Guide). You can use blue ink for the systolic BP and red ink for the heart rate.

- **Each graph will be individual and based on the interventions that the student selected.**
- **If appropriate treatment is rendered, then the trend should be a steady increase in blood pressure, while the heart rate decreases, although no progression to bradycardia occurs. Heart rate should decrease and BP increase after sodium bicarbonate and fluid bolus is given.**

12. Referring to your own graph, answer the following questions:
    a. What trends do you observe?
    b. How did your interventions relate to the trends you observe?
    c. If the trend reversed at any point, how can you explain that variation?

**Answers will vary to these questions.**

13. Complete a patient care report (PCR) for this call. (Use one of the blank PCRs in the back of your study guide or one your instructor has given you.)

**Each PCR will vary according to the treatment the student provided. Use the following guidelines to score the report. Some suggested significant information that should be noted is also included in italic print.**

**PCR Evaluation Guidelines**

| Element | Suggested Completion | Maximum Score |
|---|---|---|
| Chief complaint | Documented appropriately and completely<br>Example:<br>*Unconscious* | 1 |
| Pertinent medical history | SAMPLE history and major medical history is documented accurately.<br>Example:<br>*S—Unresponsive, lying on bathroom floor with open medication bottle near her.*<br>*A—Chocolate*<br>*M—Prenatal vitamins*<br>*P—Anorexia (hospitalized 2 months ago)*<br>*L—Ate sandwich and milk 2 hours ago.*<br>*E—Last seen at lunch. Found on bathroom floor with empty Elavil bottle (estimate 30 pills missing).* | 1 |

## PCR Evaluation Guidelines—*Continued*

| Element | Suggested Completion | Maximum Score |
|---|---|---|
| History of present illness | Events leading up to the illness or injury are clearly and concisely described in an appropriate sequence.<br><br>Example:<br><br>*Same as above and:*<br><br>*O and T—Patient was not seen for 2 hours before the call.*<br><br>*PQRS—Unknown* | 2 |
| Physical examination | Appropriate physical examination that includes pertinent negatives is documented in a clear, concise manner using appropriate medical terminology.<br><br>Example:<br><br>*Unresponsive, shallow respirations, weak, regular pulse. Breath sounds clear and equal bilaterally. Pupils midsize and react sluggishly to light. Skin color pale. Blood tinged vomit present in mouth and nose. During seizure, grinding teeth noted.* | 2 |
| Sequence and readability | The narrative is written to clearly convey the sequence of the story and includes relevant details. | 1 |
| Vital signs | Initial vital signs and those obtained after each intervention and patient change are documented accurately and completely.<br><br>NOTE: Vital signs documented should match those obtained in student log. ECG should be documented as a wide-complex supraventricular tachycardia at a rate of 134/min. | 1 |
| Interventions | Complete documentation of interventions that includes sufficient details.<br><br>*Oxygen administration, measures to clear and maintain airway, ventilation techniques, drugs with appropriate route, dose, and rate of administration. IV therapy includes volume and rate of administration. Patient positioning and other relevant interventions. Includes appropriate reassessments necessary to evaluate each intervention.* | 2 |
| Total score | | 10 |

## EXERCISE 2 ■ *Summary Activity*

Answers will vary for questions 14 through 17.

# Hematology

## ■ Assignment

### Prerequisites:

- Complete Chapter 37, Hematology, in *Mosby's Paramedic Textbook, Revised Third Edition.*
- Complete Chapter 37 in the workbook for *Mosby's Paramedic Textbook, Revised Third Edition.*
- Complete any skills or laboratory studies pertinent to this chapter.
- Read the "Getting Started" and "Orientation to Virtual Patient Encounters" sections in the *Virtual Patient Encounters Study Guide* (if this is the first lesson being attempted).

### Student assignment:

- Complete Lesson 32 in the *Virtual Patient Encounters Study Guide* after you have reviewed the topic in class.

## ■ Topic Review

### Objectives:

*On completion of this lesson, the student will be able to perform the following:*

- Interpret this patient's signs and symptoms in the context of a history of sickle cell disease.
- Discuss the pathophysiologic characteristics of sickle cell disease.
- Identify interventions needed to manage the patient's signs and symptoms.

### Review the following topics with your students before they complete the lesson:

- Hematology is the study of blood and the blood-forming organs. The paramedic must recognize the potential for alteration in normal body function when caring for patients with hematologic diseases. Management of these patients in the prehospital setting will be largely supportive and is aimed at stabilizing the patient until arrival at the emergency department.
- Sickle cell disease (sickle cell anemia) is a genetic illness that affects individuals of African and Mediterranean origin.
- Over time, the disease causes the following complications: delayed growth, jaundice, priapism, splenomegaly, and stroke.
- In sickle cells disease, an abnormal S-shaped hemoglobin is produced. In situations in which decreased oxygen is available, the S hemoglobin changes the red blood cells to a fragile, unstable sickle shape. These cells are trapped when they enter small blood vessels and impair flow to organs and tissues, causing a vasoocclusive sickle cell crisis.

- Sickle cell crisis causes pain, weakness, aching, chest pain with shortness of breath, abdominal pain, fever, and arthralgia. Over time, the crises can destroy the spleen, kidneys, gallbladder, and other organs.
- Sickle cell crisis may be triggered by dehydration, extremes in temperature, infection, lack of oxygen, physical activity, stress, or trauma.
- Three rare, but possibly life-threatening situations, may occur in sickle cell disease. In aplastic crisis, the bone marrow stops producing red blood cells. In hemolytic crisis, red blood cells break down faster than they can be replaced. In children with sickle cell disease, splenic sequestration occurs when blood becomes trapped in the spleen, causing it to enlarge, which can lead to death.
- Care of the patient with sickle cell crisis involves three key interventions: (1) oxygenation, (2) hydration, and (3) pain management.

## ■ Follow-Up

### Assignment follow-up from previous class:

- What problems, if any, did you have with your assignment?
- What questions do you have?

### In-class activities and discussion questions:

- Why do you think that some patients with sickle cell disease might be improperly labeled as drug seekers?
- Discuss several pain medications (with doses) that would be appropriate to treat a pediatric or adult patient with sickle cell crisis.

### Summary assessment:

- Administer the quiz related to this lesson (Evolve resources, instructor's test bank).

## ■ STUDY GUIDE ANSWERS

### EXERCISE 1 ■ Case 15: 42-year-old male—difficulty breathing

1. Could complications of sickle cell disease cause this patient's clinical presentation? Explain your answer.

   **Yes, patients with sickle cell disease are at higher risk for developing pulmonary emboli. The sickled red blood cells have a tendency to clump and occlude small blood vessels; they can therefore predispose the patient to clotting.**

2. What specific interventions should you perform for this patient if he has sickle cell disease?

   **Patients with sickle cell disease who have a crisis situation always need oxygen because the cells will tend to sickle in low-oxygen environments. These patients will also need intravenous fluid replacement because sickling increases in the presence of dehydration. If the patient is experiencing pain, then appropriate analgesia should be administered.**

3. Is the patient's history consistent with a situation that could cause sickle cell complications? Explain your answer.

   **The patient has been traveling and is out of his normal routine. He may have become somewhat dehydrated or perhaps has developed an infection. (Because of the damage to the spleen that occurs over time, patients with sickle cell disease are more susceptible to serious infection.) The patient should also be evaluated for pneumonia.**

4. Explain how sickle cell disease impairs his oxygen-carrying capacity before the onset of any acute illness.

   **The hemoglobin in a patient with sickle cell disease does not carry as much oxygen as normal hemoglobin. In situations in which oxygen is insufficient, the hemoglobin S crystallizes and causes the red blood cells to change to a sickle shape that can impair blood flow in small blood vessels.**

5. Explain how the red blood cells respond if oxygen is not available to them.

   **When cells do not have sufficient oxygen, they switch to anaerobic metabolism. Anaerobic metabolism produces much less energy in the form of adenosine triphosphate, and it produces the waste product, lactic acid.**

6. List signs and symptoms, which may be present in a sickle cell crisis, that are related to cellular hypoxia.

   **Signs and symptoms related to cellular hypoxia and vasooclussion in sickle cell crisis include joint pain, chest pain, weakness, shortness of breath, abdominal pain, bony deformities, and muscle aches.**

7. If this patient's vacation were in a high-altitude region, could this altitude affect his sickle cell disease? Explain your answer.

   **Yes. As altitude increases, the partial pressure of oxygen decreases. High altitude might precipitate a sickle cell crisis.**

# Environmental Conditions

## ▮ Assignment

### Prerequisites:

- Complete Chapter 38, Environmental Conditions, in *Mosby's Paramedic Textbook, Revised Third Edition.*
- Complete Chapter 38 in the workbook for *Mosby's Paramedic Textbook, Revised Third Edition.*
- Complete any skills or laboratory studies pertinent to this chapter.
- Read the "Getting Started" and "Orientation to Virtual Patient Encounters" sections in the *Virtual Patient Encounters Study Guide* (if this is the first lesson being attempted).

### Other relevant chapters:

In addition to Chapter 38, this lesson also draws content found in the following chapters:
- Chapter 10, History Taking
- Chapter 11, Techniques of Physical Examination
- Chapter 12, Patient Assessment
- Chapter 13, Clinical Decision Making
- Chapter 14, Assessment-Based Management
- Chapter 16, Documentation
- Chapter 18, Venous Access and Medication Administration
- Chapter 29, Cardiology
- Chapter 32, Endocrinology
- Chapter 49, Ambulance Operations

### Student assignment:

- Complete Lesson 33 in the *Virtual Patient Encounters Study Guide* after you have reviewed the topic in class.

## ▮ Topic Review

### Objectives:

*On completion of this lesson, the student will be able to perform the following:*

- Interpret information from the patient history and physical examination to form the appropriate clinical impression.
- Perform interventions sequentially, and revise the treatment plan based on feedback from an appropriate reassessment.

### Review the following topics with your students before they complete the lesson:

- To form the correct field impression when caring for a patient who complains of feeling weak and dizzy, the paramedic must obtain a thorough history and perform an extensive physical examination.
- This complaint may stem from an illness that originates in the heart, central nervous system, or musculoskeletal system; it may also be related to an endocrine, electrolyte, sensory, toxicologic, environmental, or behavioral abnormality.
- Cardiovascular causes may include myocardial infarction, cardiomyopathy, cardiogenic shock, or cardiac arrhythmia.
- Central nervous system causes may be related to neuromuscular disease, stroke, intracerebral lesion, infection, or a heat-related illness.
- Endocrine causes might be related to hypoglycemia associated with his diabetic history or other endocrine problems.
- Because the patient is taking a diuretic, he is susceptible to electrolyte abnormalities such as hypokalemia or hyponatremia, which can cause weakness.
- Side effects from the patient's diabetic medicine might cause acidosis. He may also be relatively dehydrated, which can predispose him to heat-related illness.
- Evaluate for the possibility of unintentional overdose causing drug toxicity or for an infectious process.
- If the temperature and humidity are high, then the patient may have a heat-related illness. This finding, coupled with the fact that he did not eat but did drink a beer, might account for the symptoms you see initially.

## ■ Follow-Up

### Assignment follow-up from previous class:

- What problems, if any, did you have with your assignment?
- What questions do you have?

### In-class activities and discussion questions:

- Ask students for examples of calls that they have been assigned during which a patient complained of feeling weak or dizzy. Discuss the causes that were identified for such symptoms in these cases.
- What physiologic changes of aging make some older patients susceptible to orthostatic dizziness?

### Other possible postcase activities:

- Have students give a radio report detailing their care of the patient.
- Ask the class or a student group to evaluate the radio report.

### Summary assessment:

- Administer the quiz related to this lesson (Evolve resources, instructor's test bank).

# ■ STUDY GUIDE ANSWERS

### EXERCISE 1 ■ *Case 12: 57-year-old male—man down*

1. What electrocardiographic (ECG) rhythm did you initially observe?

   **Sinus tachycardia.**

2. Explain the pathophysiologic cause of that rhythm.

   **Heat exhaustion can cause sinus tachycardia.**

3. Explain why you selected the oxygen device and flow rate that you did.

   **A nonrebreather mask with 12 to 15 L/min oxygen flow was selected because the patient had an increased respiratory rate and difficulty breathing, his oxygen saturation was 90%, and his skin was pale. Bag-mask ventilation would not have been appropriate at this time because the patient was alert and oriented.**

4. What noninvasive interventions should you perform before transporting? Explain the rationale for performing these interventions.

   **Noninvasive interventions for this patient would include moving him out of the sun and to a cool environment, loosening or removing excess clothes, and spraying tepid water on his skin and fanning him. Each of these interventions is aimed at reducing his body temperature without causing shivering.**

5. Identify preexisting illnesses or conditions that made this patient at high risk for his present illness. Why did these situations predispose him to this illness?

| Preexisting Condition | Rationale |
| --- | --- |
| Diabetes (takes Glucophage) | Metformin can predispose the patient to lactic acidosis. Diabetes can compromise the peripheral vasculature and impair a person's ability to vasodilate and perspire so as to compensate for increased ambient temperatures. |
| Hypertension (takes Vasotec and Bumex) | Enalapril (Vasotec) can cause dizziness and vasodilation. Bumetanide (Bumex) can cause relative depletion of water and electrolytes and predispose patients to hypotension and circulatory collapse. |
| Alcohol ingestion | Alcohol ingestion can alter blood glucose; it can also exacerbate heat-related illness. |

6. Explain the following pathophysiologic signs or symptoms and how they work to compensate for the patient's illness.

| Sign or Symptom | Mechanism of Compensation |
| --- | --- |
| Diaphoresis | **Body attempts to increase heat loss by evaporation.** |
| Respiratory rate of 32 breaths/min | **Body attempts to reduce temperature by increasing evaporative heat loss; body tries to compensate for increased metabolic needs related to increased temperature.** |

7. If you fail to intervene in a timely manner for this patient, predict the progression of his illness.

**If the condition is untreated, the patient may progress to become unconscious and develop pulmonary edema, clotting abnormalities, and cardiac dysrhythmias, causing death.**

8. If the patient begins to shiver:
   a. Explain the physiologic consequences that this sign might produce.

   **If the patient begins to shiver, then his metabolic rate and his need for oxygen will greatly increase. His heart rate and respiratory rate will increase, and his body temperature will increase from the head produced by the muscle activity during shivering. His blood glucose may also decrease.**

   b. Describe treatment measures you would use.

   **Treatment would include administration of a benzodiazepine (diazepam, lorazepam) to stop the shivering. Frequent blood glucose monitoring would also be indicated. Hypoglycemia, if present, should be treated.**

9. What environmental factors contribute to this type of illness?

**Increased ambient temperature, coupled with increased humidity contribute to the development of heat-related illness.**

10. Graph the systolic blood pressure (BP) and heart rate that you obtained in this call (consult your log). Then connect the data points so that each vital sign forms a line (see example on page 205 in the Study Guide). You can use blue ink for the systolic BP and red ink for the heart rate.
    • **Each graph will be individual and based on the interventions that the student selected.**
    • **If appropriate treatment is performed, then the systolic BP should show a steady trend upward, while the heart rate will show a steady decrease (see Chapters 7 and 11).**

11. Referring to your own graph, answer the following questions:
    a. What trends do you observe?
    b. How did your interventions relate to the trends you observed?
    c. If the trend reversed at any point, how can you explain that variation?
    **Answers will vary to these questions.**

12. Complete a patient care report (PCR) for this call. (Use one of the blank PCRs in the back of your study guide or one your instructor has given you.)

   **Each PCR will vary according to the treatment the student provided. Use the following guidelines to score the report. Some suggested significant information that should be noted is also included in italic print.**

## PCR Evaluation Guidelines

| Element | Suggested Completion | Maximum Score |
|---|---|---|
| Chief complaint | Documented appropriately and completely<br><br>**Example:**<br><br>*Weak and dizzy* | 1 |
| Pertinent medical history | SAMPLE history and major medical history is documented accurately.<br><br>**Example:**<br><br>*S—Weak, dizzy, and nauseated; diaphoretic*<br><br>*A—Morphine*<br><br>*M—Glucophage, Vasotec, Bumex*<br><br>*P—Type 2 diabetes, hypertension*<br><br>*L—Beer at clubhouse*<br><br>*E—Gradually became weak and nauseated and then became dizzy and collapsed while putting; his friend eased him to the ground; no trauma occurred.* | 1 |
| History of present illness | Events leading up to the illness or injury are clearly and concisely described in an appropriate sequence.<br><br>**Example:**<br><br>*Same as above and:*<br><br>*Onset—5 minutes before EMS call.*<br><br>*P—Nothing makes it better or worse.*<br><br>*Q—Patient says, "I can't describe it, I just feel awful. I also feel like I am going to vomit."*<br><br>*S—He denies chest pain but complains of weakness and dizziness.*<br><br>*T—5 minutes before call to EMS.* | 2 |
| Physical examination | Appropriate physical examination that includes pertinent negatives is documented in a clear, concise manner using appropriate medical terminology.<br><br>**Example:**<br><br>*Alert and oriented × 3. Respirations are labored and rapid. Breath sounds are present, clear, and equal bilaterally. Skin is pale, cool, and diaphoretic.* | 2 |

## PCR Evaluation Guidelines—*Continued*

| Element | Suggested Completion | Maximum Score |
| --- | --- | --- |
| Sequence and readability | The narrative is written to clearly convey the sequence of the story and includes relevant details. | 1 |
| Vital signs | Initial vital signs and those obtained after each intervention and patient change are documented accurately and completely.<br><br>NOTE: Vital signs documented should match those obtained in student log. ECG should be documented as sinus tachycardia. | 1 |
| Interventions | Complete documentation of interventions that includes sufficient details.<br><br>*Oxygen administration, drugs with appropriate route, dose, and rate of administration. IV therapy includes volume and rate of administration. Patient positioning and other relevant interventions. Includes appropriate reassessments necessary to evaluate each intervention.* | 2 |
| Total score | | 10 |

## EXERCISE 2 ■ *Summary Activity*

Answers will vary for questions 13 through 16.

# Infectious and Communicable Diseases

## ■ Assignment

### Prerequisites:

- Complete Chapter 39, Infectious and Communicable Diseases, in *Mosby's Paramedic Textbook, Revised Third Edition.*
- Complete Chapter 39 in the workbook for *Mosby's Paramedic Textbook, Revised Third Edition.*
- Complete any skills or laboratory studies pertinent to this chapter.
- Read the "Getting Started" and "Orientation to Virtual Patient Encounters" sections in the *Virtual Patient Encounters Study Guide* (if this is the first lesson being attempted).

### Student assignment:

- Complete Lesson 34 in the *Virtual Patient Encounters Study Guide* after you have reviewed the topic in class.

## ■ Topic Review

### Objectives:

*On completion of this lesson, the student will be able to perform the following:*

- Recognize appropriate personal protective equipment to prevent infectious disease exposure on selected cases.
- Outline how the chain of disease transmission relates to tuberculosis.
- Identify medications used to treat infectious diseases.
- Discuss actions that should be taken after exposure to blood or body fluids.

### Review the following topics with your students before they complete the lesson:

- Emergencies related to infectious and communicable diseases are common in the prehospital setting. Paramedics must recognize patients who pose a risk of transmission of infectious disease and take measures to minimize the risk of exposure or transmission of these diseases.
- Use standard precautions on all calls. In addition, wash your hands, or clean them with an alcohol-based waterless cleanser each time you remove your gloves or if your hands become soiled. If a waterless cleanser is used, wash your hands as soon as soap and water are available.
- Follow departmental equipment decontamination guidelines. Equipment should be cleaned using sterilization, high-level, intermediate, or low-level disinfection. Use the appropriate level of disinfection based on the nature of the equipment and level of contamination.

- The chain of transmission of infectious disease must be intact for disease to spread. The chain includes the pathogenic agent, reservoir, portal of exit, transmission, portal of entry, and host susceptibility. Paramedics should use measures to interrupt the chain so that infectious disease transmission is stopped.

- External barriers to prevent infection include flora, the skin, the gastrointestinal system, the upper respiratory tract, and the genitourinary tract.

- Internal barriers to infection include the inflammatory response and the immune response. The inflammatory response includes the cellular response to injury, vascular response to injury, and phagocytosis.

- Infection with a disease follows four distinct stages: (1) latent period, (2) incubation period, (3) communicability period, and (4) disease period. During the latent period, the person is infected but cannot infect others. The incubation period is the time between exposure and onset of symptoms of disease. During the communicable period, the disease can be spread to others. The disease period follows the incubation period.

- If you have a significant exposure, then you must report it immediately to the appropriate personnel so a determination can be made whether any postexposure prophylaxis is possible. The exposure should be reported to the designated officer for infectious disease at your agency, as well as to a nurse or physician who is caring for the patient at the receiving facility. Follow your departmental exposure policy.

- After significant exposure to some diseases or to a high-risk patient, postexposure prophylaxis with drugs or immune globulin may be indicated. The health care provider who is caring for you should explain the risks and benefits of postexposure treatment so you can make an informed decision to take or refuse the medicines. Additionally, initial and follow-up blood tests may be performed to determine if you become infected with the disease.

# ■ Follow-Up

### Assignment follow-up from previous class:

- What problems, if any, did you have with your assignment?
- What questions do you have?

### In-class activities and discussion questions:

- Spray some liquid that contains a fluorescent substance such as Glo Germ™ into the back of an ambulance (or classroom). Use a fluorescent light to see how far the spray traveled, and then discuss why PPE is important to prevent splash or spray or airborne contamination.
- Ask a health care provider who has, in the past, been exposed to a high-risk patient to come and talk about the decision to take postexposure drugs, the side effects of the drugs, and the emotional effects of a high-risk exposure.

### Other possible postcase activities:

- Have students give a radio report detailing their care of the patient.
- Ask the class or a student group to evaluate the radio report.

### Summary assessment:

- Administer the quiz related to this lesson (Evolve resources, instructor's test bank).

# ■ STUDY GUIDE ANSWERS

### EXERCISE 1 ■ *Case 15: 42-year-old male—difficulty breathing*

1. Explain how tuberculosis can be spread by identifying how its characteristics relate to each link in the chain of transmission of infection.

| Link | Tuberculosis |
|---|---|
| Pathogenic agent | Bacteria (*Mycobacterium tuberculosis, Mycobacterium bovis*) |
| Reservoir | Usually the lungs |
| Portal of exit | Airborne droplets or sputum |
| Transmission | Airborne (respiratory) or, rarely, contact |
| Portal of entry | Usually nose or mouth |
| Host susceptibility | If general state of health of exposed person is poor, then the risk of infection is increased. |

2. If you suspect that a patient is infectious with pulmonary tuberculosis, what measures should you take to prevent exposure during the care and transport of this patient?

   **Apply a surgical mask to the patient. Rescuers should wear an N-95 or high-efficiency particulate air (HEPA) filter mask. Use HEPA ventilation system or nonrecirculation ventilation in ambulance.**

3. How should you clean the ambulance after the call?

   **Clean surfaces in ambulance with a disinfectant. The label should specify that the disinfectant is tuberculocidal.**

4. Do you think this patient's acute signs and symptoms presented in this case are related to tuberculosis? Explain your answer.

   **The patient's signs and symptoms are unlikely to be related to tuberculosis. He does not report cough, and he states he has been told he is not contagious; he reports sudden onset of dyspnea and aching in chest.**

5. Which of the patient's home medicines are used to treat tuberculosis?

   **Rifamate (Rifampin)**

6. List at least two other medications that may be used to treat tuberculosis.

   **Pyrazinamide, ethambutol, streptomycin, isoniazid**

7. If you were to be exposed to tuberculosis on this call and your purified protein derivative (PPD) skin test in 6 months is positive, identify the following characteristics of prophylactic isoniazid, the drug you will likely take to prevent illness related to tuberculosis.

| Drug | Should Avoid | Side Effects |
|------|------|------|
| Isoniazid | **Alcohol, pregnancy** | **Hepatitis, paresthesias, seizures, orthostatic hypotension, nausea, vomiting, hypersensitivity** |

**EXERCISE 2 ■ *Case 5: 40-year-old male—vomiting blood***

8. What diseases present a high risk of exposure on this call?

   **The patient is vomiting large amounts of blood, which may expose the paramedics by splash or spray, possibly leading to exposure to hepatitis B or C or human immunodeficiency virus infection (HIV) infection.**

9. What measures should the crew take to prevent significant exposure on this call?

   **The crew should wear gloves, gown, and face shield (including nose, mouth, eye protection).**

10. Which of the following situations might represent a reportable significant exposure to blood or bloody body fluids on this call? What actions should you take before you report the exposure?

| Situation | Significant? (Yes or No) | Immediate Actions Needed |
|------|------|------|
| Patient vomits, and you are certain that some of the vomit got into your eyes. | **Yes** | **Wash your face off and irrigate your eyes as soon as possible using normal saline (or tap water).** |
| A lancet barely pierces the skin on your thumb after assessing the level of blood glucose of the patient. You do not see any any blood. | **Yes** | **Clean your hands with soap and water or waterless hand cleanser (until hand washing can be performed) as soon as possible.** |
| When you arrive at the hospital, you notice some blood smeared on the intact skin of your forearm. | **No** | **Wash the area thoroughly with soap and water.** |
| While cleaning the ambulance after the call, an intravenous (IV) needle, which fell to the floor while this patient's IV was being started, sticks you. It is bleeding. | **Yes** | **Wash the area thoroughly with soap and water or waterless hand cleanser (until soap and water is available) as soon as possible.** |

11. Which of the significant exposures you identified in the previous question present the highest risk?

   **The needle stick with the contaminated IV needle is the highest risk for exposure.**

12. What history or physical findings would identify a patient as being at particularly high risk for an infectious disease?

   **History of infectious disease (HIV, hepatitis), needle track marks, or reported history of IV drug use or known high risk behaviors (e.g., prostitution) are all indicators that the patient is at high risk for infection with a communicable disease.**

13. Answer the following questions related to follow-up if you had a significant exposure on this call.

   a. To whom should you report this exposure?

   **This incident should be reported according to your agency's protocols and policies. Minimally, the exposure should be reported to your designated officer for infectious disease and to a nurse or physician who is responsible for the patient's care at the receiving facility.**

   b. When should you report this exposure?

   **It should be reported immediately, as soon as emergency patient care has concluded.**

14. Identify the specific postexposure prophylaxis (PEP) that is available for each of the following infectious diseases:

| Disease | Postexposure Prophylaxis |
| --- | --- |
| Human immunodeficiency virus | **Depending on the patient risk and source patient test results; may include zidovudine or lamivudine.** |
| Hepatitis B (HBV) | **Source test for antibodies against HBV. If not previously vaccinated against HBV or antibody titer is low, then administer hepatitis B immune globulin following by HBV vaccination.** |
| Hepatitis C (HCV) | **The Centers for Disease Control and Prevention recommends no postexposure prophylaxis at this time.** |

# Behavioral and Psychiatric Disorders

## ■ Assignment

### Prerequisites:

- Complete Chapter 40, Behavioral and Psychiatric Disorders, in *Mosby's Paramedic Textbook, Revised Third Edition.*
- Complete Chapter 40 in the workbook for *Mosby's Paramedic Textbook, Revised Third Edition.*
- Complete any skills or laboratory studies pertinent to this chapter.
- Read the "Getting Started" and "Orientation to Virtual Patient Encounters" sections in the *Virtual Patient Encounters Study Guide* (if this is the first lesson being attempted).

### Other relevant chapters:

In addition to Chapter 40, this lesson also draws content found in the following chapters:
- Chapter 2, The Well-Being of the Paramedic
- Chapter 4, Medical/Legal Issues
- Chapter 5, Ethics
- Chapter 10, History Taking
- Chapter 11, Techniques of Physical Examination
- Chapter 12, Patient Assessment
- Chapter 16, Documentation
- Chapter 17, Pharmacology
- Chapter 18, Venous Access and Medication Administration
- Chapter 19, Airway Management and Ventilation

### Student assignment:

- Complete Lesson 35 in the *Virtual Patient Encounters Study Guide* after you have reviewed the topic in class.

## ■ Topic Review

### Objectives:

*On completion of this lesson, the student will be able to perform the following:*
- Demonstrate knowledge of the appropriate techniques to restrain a patient physically or chemically.
- Describe appropriate measures to monitor a restrained patient.
- Anticipate problems that can occur when a patient is restrained.

- Outline techniques to distinguish medical versus psychiatric causes of behavioral illness.
- Identify selected medications used to treat patients with behavioral illness.
- State appropriate techniques to use to communicate with a patient with a behavioral emergency.

***Review the following topics with your students before they complete the lesson:***

- The first consideration on any behavioral call should be the safety of the responding crew. Ensure that you have an adequate response with appropriate supporting agencies to care safely for your patient.
- Patients with a psychiatric emergency have some type of abnormal behavior that deviates from societal norms, interferes with the patient's ability to function, or harms the individual or others.
- Behavioral emergencies can be related to biologic, psychosocial, or sociocultural causes.
- Prehospital providers must have several priorities:
    1. Ensure safety of the crew and the patient.
    2. Rule out treatable physical causes.
    3. Manage the behavior of the patient to allow for safe transport.
- Once physical causes of the behavioral illness have been ruled out, focus on identifying the patient's concerns and on managing his or her behavior.
- Good communication skills are usually the only intervention needed en route to the hospital. Conveying a calm, caring, accepting demeanor is often sufficient to allow a safe transport to occur without incident.
- In the rare event that you are legally permitted to transport a patient against his or her wishes, and you must use restraints to accomplish this task safely; strict precautions should be observed.
- All actions involving the restraint should be performed while keeping in mind the therapeutic benefit of the intervention. The patient should be informed of planned actions and treated with dignity.
- Physical restraint should be preplanned and performed in a manner that minimizes risk of injury to patients or caregivers.
- Chemical restraint may also be ordered and will vary according to local protocols.
- Guidelines should be in place for monitoring the patient who is restrained to ensure that any change in condition is identified quickly and to address the physical needs of the patient during transport. Measures to release the patient's restraints quickly in the event of sudden physical deterioration should be in place.

# Follow-Up

***Assignment follow-up from previous class:***

- What problems, if any, did you have with your assignment?
- What questions do you have?

***In-class activities and discussion questions:***

- What is the particular importance of considering what you will say to this patient during your initial contact with him?
- What will you do if the police place the patient in prone restraint and refuse to assist you to move him?
- Why is continuously monitoring a patient who is restrained essential?

*Other possible postcase activities:*
- Have students give a radio report detailing their care of the patient.
- Ask the class or a student group to evaluate the radio report.

*Summary assessment:*
- Administer the quiz related to this lesson (Evolve resources, instructor's test bank).

# ■ STUDY GUIDE ANSWERS

### EXERCISE 1 ■ *Case 8: 38-year-old male—suicide attempt*

1. Why should you stage and not approach the scene on this type of dispatch until the police signal that the scene is safe?

   **A person wishing to harm himself or herself may display violence towards others; or, the patient may have an altered sense of reality and hurt rescuers without intending to do so. Stage at a safe distance until police arrive and secure the scene.**

2. How did the police place the patient on the stretcher?

   **Police placed the patient on the stretcher prone, with his arms and legs cuffed behind him (hog-tied).**

3. Is leaving the patient restrained in that manner acceptable to you? Explain your answer.

   **No. Leaving the patient restrained in this manner can be dangerous and is reported to have contributed to patient deaths, especially when the patient is intoxicated with hallucinogens or stimulants. This type of restraint is thought to impair ventilation and may cause sudden cardiac death; therefore it is not an acceptable manner to restrain a patient. He should be moved to a supine position and properly restrained immediately.**

4. Were the police officer's initial comments to the patient appropriate? Explain your answer.

   **The police officer communicated to him in a kind manner, was very direct about his expectations (move away from the ledge), and told the patient that the officer was there to help him. The officer's comments were appropriate under the circumstances.**

5. What type of abnormal communication did you observe this patient make?

   **The patient displayed disorganized thoughts and flight of ideas—his speech was rambling and often disconnected. He appeared paranoid and delusional.**

6. Could you predict at least two behavioral illnesses he might have? List three medications that he might be taking for each condition you listed and the side effect associated with each medication.

| Behavioral Illness | Medications | Side Effects |
|---|---|---|
| Schizophrenia | Antipsychotic agents: chlorpromazine (Thorazine), thioridazine (Mellaril), fluphenazine (Prolixin), haloperidol (Haldol), molindone (Moban), loxapine (Loxitane), olanzapine (Zyprexa), clozapine (Clozaril), risperidone (Risperdal) | Dyskinesia |
| Bipolar disorder with mania | Lithium | Muscle tremors, increased thirst, nausea, polyuria, abdominal cramps, diarrhea |
| | Selective serotonin reuptake inhibitors: fluoxetine (Prozac), sertraline (Zoloft), paroxetine (Paxil), fluvoxamine (Luvox), citalopram (Celexa) | Insomnia, difficulty with orgasm |
| | Tricyclic antidepressants: mirtazapine (Remeron), nortriptyline (Pamelor), amitriptyline (Elavil) | Dry mouth, difficulty concentrating |

7. During your assessment of this patient, you will need to rule out any organic cause of his bizarre behavior. List at least six possible organic causes of altered mental status and one or two specific signs or symptoms that you will assess to rule out these causes.

| Organic Cause | Signs or Symptoms to Assess |
|---|---|
| Diabetic problems (hypoglycemia or hyperglycemia) | Check blood glucose level. |
| Head injury | Assess for any trauma to the head; perform neurologic examination to check for focal neurologic findings. |
| Stroke | Assess using the Cincinnati Stroke Scale. |
| Toxic ingestion or drug or alcohol abuse | Assess for any evidence of drug overdose. Check pupil size and reactivity. Look for illicit drug paraphernalia on patient. Note odors such as alcohol or marijuana on patient's breath. |
| Intracranial lesion | Assess for focal nerve deficits, cranial nerve function. |
| Other metabolic disorders | Check for edema and uremic frost associated with advanced renal failure. Also check for jaundice, electrocardiographic changes, and enlarged liver associated with advanced liver failure. |
| Infectious diseases | Assess for fever, nuchal rigidity, petechial rash, and septic shock. |

8. List at least two alternate drugs that you could have administered in this case. Include the drug classes, doses and routes of administration, and side effects you should anticipate. If the drug can be given intravenously (IV), then specify how fast you will administer it.

| Drug | Class | Dose and Route | Possible Side Effects |
| --- | --- | --- | --- |
| Diazepam | Benzodiazepine | 5 mg IV over 2 min | Hypotension, ataxia, respiratory depression, psychomotor impairment, confusion, nausea |
| Lorazepam | Benzodiazepine | 1-4 mg IV or IM over 2-10 min | Hypotension, ataxia, respiratory depression, psychomotor impairment, confusion, tachycardia, bradycardia |
| Midazolam | Benzodiazepine | 1-2.5 mg IV or IM over 2-4 min | Respiratory depression or arrest, hiccup, cough, oversedation, pain at injection site, nausea, vomiting, blurred vision, hypotension, headache |
| Haloperidol | Antipsychotic neuroleptic | 2-5 mg IM | Extrapyramidal reactions, hypotension, nausea, vomiting, allergic reactions, blurred vision. |

9. What nonpharmacologic measures can you take to calm this patient's behavior during your care and transportation?

**Talk to the patient in a calm, quiet voice. Minimize sensory stimulation (lower lights; do not use lights or siren if the patient's condition remains stable).**

10. What specific patient assessment is necessary for a patient who is restrained?

**Assess respiratory function (respiratory rate and oxygen saturation) and circulatory function (heart rate, blood pressure, and pulse, as well as movement and sensation in all extremities) at least every 5 to 10 minutes. Document these assessments.**

11. Complete a patient care report (PCR) for this call. (Use one of the blank PCRs in the back of your study guide or one your instructor has given you.)

**Each PCR will vary according to the treatment the student provided. Use the following guidelines to score the report. Some suggested significant information that should be noted is also included in italic print.**

## PCR Evaluation Guidelines

| Element | Suggested Completion | Maximum Score |
| --- | --- | --- |
| Chief complaint | Documented appropriately and completely Example: *Attempted suicide* | 1 |

**PCR Evaluation Guidelines**—*Continued*

| Element | Suggested Completion | Maximum Score |
|---|---|---|
| Pertinent medical history | SAMPLE history and major medical history is documented accurately.<br><br>Example:<br><br>*S—Alert, but not oriented*<br><br>*A—Unknown*<br><br>*M—Takes unknown medicine. His friend states that his behavior becomes bizarre when he does not take it.*<br><br>*P—Unknown behavioral illness*<br><br>*L—Unknown*<br><br>*E—Was passenger in a car. Tried to get out of the moving vehicle. Friend stopped the car, and the patient ran off into the woods, stopped at the edge of the cliff, and started to yell incoherent phrases. Friend was unable to "talk him out of it."* | 1 |
| History of present illness | Events leading up to the illness or injury are clearly and concisely described in an appropriate sequence.<br><br>Example:<br><br>*Same as above and:*<br><br>*O—Approximately 5 minutes before calling EMS*<br><br>*P—Patient stopped taking his medication.*<br><br>*Q—Delusional and suicidal*<br><br>*R—Unknown*<br><br>*S—Patient is a threat to himself and possibly others.*<br><br>*T—Approximately 5 minutes before the call to EMS* | 2 |
| Physical examination | Appropriate physical examination that includes pertinent negatives is documented in a clear, concise manner using appropriate medical terminology.<br><br>Example:<br><br>*Awake and alert but not oriented to person, place, or time. Pupils are midsize and reactive to light. Skin is warm and flushed. Breath sounds are clear and equal bilaterally. No apparent injuries or abnormalities identified in focused examination.* | 2 |

## PCR Evaluation Guidelines—*Continued*

| Element | Suggested Completion | Maximum Score |
|---|---|---|
| Sequence and readability | The narrative is written to clearly convey the sequence of the story and includes relevant details. | 1 |
| Vital signs | Initial vital signs and those obtained after each intervention and patient change are documented accurately and completely. | 1 |
| | NOTE: Vital signs documented should match those obtained in student log. | |
| Interventions | Complete documentation of interventions that includes sufficient details. | 2 |
| | *Drugs with appropriate route, dose, and rate of administration. IV therapy includes volume and rate of administration. Patient positioning and specifics as to how the patient was restrained. Includes appropriate reassessments necessary to evaluate each intervention.* | |
| Total score | | 10 |

## EXERCISE 2 ■ *Summary Activity*

Answers will vary for questions 12 through 15.

# Gynecology

## ■ Assignment

### Prerequisites:

- Complete Chapter 41, Gynecology, in *Mosby's Paramedic Textbook, Revised Third Edition.*
- Complete Chapter 41 in the workbook for *Mosby's Paramedic Textbook, Revised Third Edition.*
- Complete any skills or laboratory studies pertinent to this chapter.
- Read the "Getting Started" and "Orientation to Virtual Patient Encounters" sections in the *Virtual Patient Encounters Study Guide* (if this is the first lesson being attempted).

### Student assignment:

- Complete Lesson 36 in the *Virtual Patient Encounters Study Guide* after you have reviewed the topic in class.

## ■ Topic Review

### Objectives:

*On completion of this lesson, the student will be able to perform the following:*

- Describe how emotional response to a sexual assault can affect taking the patient's history.
- Identify gynecologic problems that can result in shock.
- Describe how to integrate evidence collection into the assessment and management of a patient who was sexually assaulted.

### Review the following topics with your students before they complete the lesson:

- Sexual assault is a violent crime that can inflict serious physical and emotional injuries.
- The initial priority when caring for a patient who has been sexually assaulted is to identify and manage any life-threatening injuries that may be present.
- Privacy during the patient interview and examination is critical. If possible, the patient should be examined and treated by a paramedic of the same gender.
- History taking related to the event should be limited to asking patient questions that relate directly to emergency care. Questions that are specific to the sexual assault itself should generally be postponed until arrival at the emergency department.
- Emotional reactions to sexual assault will vary according to the individual and the nature of the attack. The patient may be silent, anxious, angry, in denial, or fearful.
- Limit physical assessment to general assessment for the presence of serious or life-threatening injuries. The genitalia should be examined only if serious injury needing immediate care is present or strongly suggested. Explain all procedures before you perform them.

- Paramedics should adopt a nonjudgmental attitude related to the patient and the history of the assault. Maintaining a professional attitude is important.
- Paramedics should convey that the patient will be safe during transport. Provide emotional support, and facilitate a supportive environment if the patient chooses to talk about the assault.
- Other gynecologic emergencies can cause life-threatening illness and shock. These emergencies include rupture of an ovarian cyst or ectopic pregnancy rupture. Pain is often unilateral and severe and may radiate to the shoulder. The patient should be questioned about her last menstrual period and the presence of vaginal bleeding. Monitor vital signs closely, anticipate shock, and provide rapid transport.

# ■ Follow-Up

## Assignment follow-up from previous class:

- What problems, if any, did you have with your assignment?
- What questions do you have?

## In-class activities and discussion questions:

- Ask the class members why they think some people have a bias toward a patient who says she has been sexually assaulted.
- How can you distinguish a gynecologic condition that is nonemergent from one that has the potential to cause shock and/or death?

## Other possible postcase activities:

- Have students give a radio report detailing their care of the patient.
- Ask the class or a student group to evaluate the radio report.

## Summary assessment:

- Administer the quiz related to this lesson (Evolve resources, instructor's test bank).

# ■ STUDY GUIDE ANSWERS

### EXERCISE 1 ■ Case 9: 22-year-old female—assault

1. Describe the patient's emotional response to the assault.

   **She appears to be fearful and sad. She is reluctant to speak; however, this reluctance may be related to her other injuries or to any drugs that she was given while in captivity.**

2. What other responses might you anticipate from a person who has been sexually assaulted?

   **Denial and anger are two other possible responses.**

3. How might you adapt your assessment and management of this patient to assist the patient emotionally?

   **Allow her to speak openly. Explain all procedures and examination techniques before using them. If a female paramedic is present, allow her to be the primary caregiver, if possible. In this case, allow the female law enforcement officer to remain with the patient. Do not verbalize judgments or responses to the patient's statements.**

4. List the priorities in assessment and care of this patient.

**The first priority is to perform an initial assessment to find and treat any life-threatening injuries that may be present. If bleeding from the vagina or rectum occurred, the perineum would be examined to assess and control bleeding. If not, the gynecologic examination should be postponed until the patient reaches the hospital.**

5. What actions can you take or instruct the patient to take to preserve any evidence associated with the alleged assault?

**Evidence preservation can be enhanced by the following actions. Handle the patient's clothing as little as possible. If clothing must be removed, place each item in a separate bag (not plastic if clothing is wet with blood or other fluid). If possible, do not clean wounds. The patient should be instructed not to drink, eat, or brush teeth. Tell the patient not to bathe or change clothes. If the patient is found at the scene of the crime, avoid disturbing the scene.**

6. How can you document your findings and the patient's statements to ensure that they will be legally defensible if introduced as evidence in the assault trial?

**You should document all examination findings, including observations related to the patient's emotional state. Note anything unusual in the environment. Include any relevant statements made by the patient or others on the scene. Document objectively. Record statements in the patient's words and place them in quotes. Avoid opinions in your documentation.**

7. What injuries should you anticipate related to the sexual assault of a female patient?

**Vaginal or rectal lacerations or tearing that can result in significant bleeding.**

## EXERCISE 2 ■ Case 6: 16-year-old female—unknown medical

8. What gynecologic emergencies could cause this patient's signs and symptoms?

**Shock related to ruptured ovarian cyst, ectopic pregnancy, or an infection that has caused sepsis**

9. If this patient were conscious, what questions would you ask to determine whether a gynecologic problem is the cause of her emergency?

**When was her last menstrual cycle, if she reached menarche? If she has pain, what is the history of that pain (location, severity, radiation), is she sexually active, does she have vaginal bleeding or discharge, and has she had a fever?**

10. At what age do most women reach menarche?

**Women reach menarche at 12 to 13 years of age.**

11. Can you identify a possible reason why this patient may not yet have reached menarche?

**Low body weight associated with anorexia can result in delayed menarche.**

# Obstetrics

## ■ Assignment

### *Prerequisites:*

- Complete Chapter 42, Obstetrics, in *Mosby's Paramedic Textbook, Revised Third Edition.*
- Complete Chapter 42 in the workbook for *Mosby's Paramedic Textbook, Revised Third Edition.*
- Complete any skills or laboratory studies pertinent to this chapter.
- Read the "Getting Started" and "Orientation to Virtual Patient Encounters" sections in the *Virtual Patient Encounters Study Guide* (if this is the first lesson being attempted).

### *Other relevant chapters:*

In addition to Chapter 42, this lesson also draws content found in the following chapters:
- Chapter 9, Therapeutic Communication
- Chapter 10, History Taking
- Chapter 11, Techniques of Physical Examination
- Chapter 16, Documentation
- Chapter 17, Pharmacology
- Chapter 18, Venous Access and Mediation Administration
- Chapter 19, Airway Management and Ventilation
- Chapter 31, Neurology

### *Student assignment:*

- Complete Lesson 37 in the *Virtual Patient Encounters Study Guide* after you have reviewed the topic in class.

## ■ Topic Review

### *Objectives:*

*On completion of this lesson, the student will be able to perform the following:*
- Recognize and treat the complications of pregnancy.
- Anticipate signs and symptoms that may develop in a patient with complications of pregnancy.
- Demonstrate management of seizures in a pregnant patient.
- Anticipate the effects of interventions to manage complications of pregnancy.

### Review the following topics with your students before they complete the lesson:

- Assessment of the pregnant patient can be complex and involve a high-risk situation that affects not only one patient, but two patients. During pregnancy, considering the effects of the injury or illness on the patient and on the fetus is important.

- First, determine the patient's chief complaint. Assess to see if the complaint is related to the pregnancy or if it might affect the pregnancy. Then, obtain a history of the pregnancy.

- Initial pregnancy history should include the following:

  1. How long she has been pregnant

  2. Number of pregnancies (gravida) the patient has had

  3. Number of pregnancies that were carried to term (para).

- Also inquire about infectious disease or previous complications related to the patient's gynecologic or obstetrical history.

- If abdominal pain is present, determine when it started, the character, duration, location, and radiation of the pain.

- Determine if vaginal discharge or bleeding is present. If so, then the quantity and color should be noted. Also note any vaginal discharge and whether the patient has bloody show or if membranes have ruptured.

- Determine the general health of the mother, ask if she is allergic to medicines or takes any medicine (or alcohol or recreational drugs), and inquire about any other medical conditions. Find out if she is receiving routine prenatal care.

- If the patient has abdominal pain, then determine if the pain is related to labor. Time the contractions, if present, and ask the mother if she has the urge to bear down or feels as though she has to have a bowel movement. Check the perineum for crowning if you believe that delivery is imminent.

- If you have the proper equipment, assess the fetal health by listening to fetal heart tones. Abnormal fetal heart tones can indicate fetal distress. You can also ask the mother if she has felt fetal movement since this illness or trauma occurred and whether fetal movement is normal.

- If a condition is identified that has the potential to harm the mother or fetus, administer high-flow oxygen and transport the patient immediately in the left lateral recumbent position to the closest appropriate medical facility.

# ■ Follow-Up

### Assignment follow-up from previous class:

- What problems, if any, did you have with your assignment?

- What questions do you have?

### In-class activities and discussion questions:

- Obtain a Doppler ultrasound device or fetoscope (or both) and demonstrate how to auscultate fetal heart tones.

- Discuss effective measures to monitor for respiratory depression if magnesium sulfate is given (capnography and oxygen saturation).

### Other possible postcase activities:

- Have students give a radio report detailing their care of the patient.

- Ask the class or a student group to evaluate the radio report.

*Summary assessment:*

• Administer the quiz related to this lesson (Evolve resources, instructor's test bank).

# ■ STUDY GUIDE ANSWERS

### EXERCISE 1 ■ *Case 10: 25-year-old female—abdominal pain*

1. What communication barrier did you encounter on this call?

   **The patient was Hispanic, and the information related to the history and examination of the patient had to be relayed through an interpreter. This circumstance can increase the time on the scene and can result in misinterpretation of information.**

2. How would you have handled this barrier if the patient's friend were not present on the call?

   **If no interpreter were on the scene, then critical information might have been missed on this call. The patient's signs and symptoms might have been misinterpreted, which may have affected her care. If a translator is not available, consider using a translation device. Many of these devices are available on the market; some of them require you to say and interpret key phrases, whereas others are more universal and have pictures to which you and the patient can point for communication. In some systems, telephonic translation services will be available.**

3. Explain why you selected the oxygen device and flow rate that you did.

   **High-flow oxygen should be selected because, even though the mother's oxygen saturation level was initially within normal limits, her condition can cause diminished blood flow to her fetus. In any situation in which any possibility exists of decreased placental blood flow, the highest amount of oxygen possible must be administered.**

4. What additional physical findings might you observe that would confirm your initial clinical impression of this patient?

   **Assess for confusion, double vision, nausea and vomiting, reduced urine output or blood in the urine, and fetal distress.**

5. Describe the pathophysiologic causes of the signs and symptoms you observed in the patient on this call.

| Sign or Symptom | Pathophysiologic Cause |
| --- | --- |
| Blood pressure (BP) 150/98 mm Hg | **Hypertension is related to vasospasm.** |
| Rash on abdomen | **Activation of the clotting cascade has occurred.** |
| Edema | **Increased capillary permeability allows blood to leak into the interstitial spaces.** |

6. Transporting this patient involves important considerations.

   a. List two acceptable positions for this patient during transport:

   **She may be transported in a Fowler position if she is conscious and alert; if she is lying flat, transport in the left lateral recumbent position.**

   b. Discuss measures that should be taken for supportive care of this patient during transport:

   **Environmental stimuli should be kept to a minimum. Unless her condition deteriorates, no lights and sirens should be used.**

   c. Describe how you might determine the appropriate transport destination for this patient:

   **If a specialty obstetrical center is located immediately within your transport area, she should be taken there because she will likely have to have an emergency cesarean section, and the baby may need resuscitation and specialty services.**

7. This patient has severe abdominal pain.

   a. What is a possible life-threatening cause of this pain?

   **Abruptio placenta is a possible complication of preeclampsia.**

   b. What signs and symptoms related to her pain will you assess for?

   **You should observe for signs of shock, fetal distress, abdominal pain, and vaginal bleeding, which may or may not be present in abruptio.**

   c. What are the implications of the cause of this pain to the mother and fetus?

   **Abruptio placenta can cause life-threatening hemorrhage and death of the mother; it can also cause fetal death resulting from hypoxia.**

8. Describe how you might assess fetal heart tones (FHTs) on this patient.

   **The most likely site for fetal heart tone auscultation at this stage of pregnancy would be lateral to the umbilicus toward the mother's left side. A fetoscope or Doppler ultrasound equipment may be used. If heart tones are not audible in this location, then listen slightly inferior or on the other side.**

9. You have assessed FHTs on this patient, and you observe the following findings. Discuss the significance of each finding.

| Initial FHT | Significance |
| --- | --- |
| 100 bpm | **This finding represents fetal bradycardia and indicates severe fetal distress. Oxygenate the mother, lay her down in the left lateral recumbent position, and transport urgently to the closest appropriate facility.** |
| 140 bpm | **This finding is within the normal range of fetal heart tones. Continue monitoring during transport.** |
| 200 bpm | **This finding represents fetal tachycardia. It may be a temporary increase associated with movement of the baby, or it may indicate distress. Re-evaluate often, and, if unchanged, oxygenate the mother, lay her down in the left lateral recumbent position, and transport urgently to the closest appropriate facility.** |

10. If this patient were to have a seizure, all of the benzodiazepines have a pregnancy category "D."

    a. Describe what a pregnancy category "D" means:

    **Pregnancy category D means that evidence exists of fetal harm if this drug is given. However, the benefits of administration may be acceptable despite the risk if a safer drug is not available.**

    b. Discuss how this category would affect your care:

    **If this patient has a seizure, then benzodiazepines with a category D rating will be administered because they are essential to stop the seizure.**

11. List at least three drugs with appropriate doses and routes (including one that is not a benzodiazepine) that would be indicated to treat seizure activity in the patient.

| Trade Name | Generic Name | Dose and Route |
|---|---|---|
| Ativan | Lorazepam | 1-4 mg IV or IM |
| Valium | Diazepam | 5 mg over 2 min IV |
| Versed | Midazolam | 1.0-2.5 mg IV or IM |
| Not applicable | Magnesium sulfate | 1-4 g IV infusion |

*IM,* Intramuscular; *IV,* intravenous.

12. Complete a patient care report (PCR) for this call. (Use one of the blank PCR in the back of your study guide or one your instructor has given you.)

**Each PCR will vary according to the treatment the student provided. Use the following guidelines to score the report. Some suggested significant information that should be noted is also included in italic print.**

**PCR Evaluation Guidelines**

| Element | Suggested Completion | Maximum Score |
|---|---|---|
| Chief complaint | Documented appropriately and completely<br>Example:<br>  *Abdominal pain* | 1 |
| Pertinent medical history | SAMPLE history and major medical history is documented accurately.<br>Example:<br>*S—Gravida 3 Para 0; two miscarriages. Prenatal care for the first 5 months of the pregnancy. Has not had prenatal care for 3 months. Has "1 month to go" in pregnancy.*<br>*A—Denies*<br>*M—Prenatal vitamins*<br>*P—Has not felt well for 3 weeks. No energy, headaches, leg aches, and cramps.* | 1 |

### PCR Evaluation Guidelines—*Continued*

| Element | Suggested Completion | Maximum Score |
|---------|----------------------|:-------------:|
| | *L—Ate breakfast.* | |
| | *E—Swelling for 3 weeks but has worsened this week. Abdominal pain began last night. Is dizzy when walking today. "Can't see straight" (blurred vision). Light hurts her eyes. Denies vaginal discharge or that her water broke. No pushing observed. Found by neighbor on couch with washcloth over her eyes.* | |
| History of present illness | Events leading up to the illness or injury are clearly and concisely described in an appropriate sequence.<br><br>**Example:**<br><br>*Same as above and:*<br><br>*O—Pain began last night.*<br><br>*P—Pain is less when she lies still. Walking increases the pain. Light hurts her eyes.*<br><br>*Q—Pain is a constant, deep ache.*<br><br>*R—Pain radiates to low back.*<br><br>*S—9/10*<br><br>*T—Pain is increasing steadily since last night.* | 2 |
| Physical examination | Appropriate physical examination that includes pertinent negatives is documented in a clear, concise manner using appropriate medical terminology.<br><br>**Example:**<br><br>*Respirations are shallow; pulse is regular and strong; pupils are midsize, equal, and reactive; facial twitching and periorbital and facial edema are present. Lung sounds are clear and equal to auscultation. Skin is pink, warm, and dry. Fine, petechial rash noted on lateral aspects of abdomen. Fundal height is 2 fingerbreadths below xiphoid process. Abdomen is tense. No contractions palpated; hands swollen, pitting edema from foot to mid-shin bilaterally; no abnormalities noted on perineal examination. Hyperreflexia is noted in upper and lower extremities.* | 2 |
| Sequence and readability | The narrative is written to clearly convey the sequence of the story and includes relevant details. | 1 |

**PCR Evaluation Guidelines**—*Continued*

| Element | Suggested Completion | Maximum Score |
|---|---|---|
| Vital signs | Initial vital signs and those obtained after each intervention and patient change are documented accurately and completely.<br><br>NOTE: Vital signs documented should match those obtained in student log. | 1 |
| Interventions | Complete documentation of interventions that includes sufficient details.<br><br>*Oxygen administration, drugs with appropriate route, dose, and rate of administration. IV therapy includes volume and rate of administration. Patient positioning and other relevant interventions. Includes appropriate reassessments necessary to evaluate each intervention.* | 2 |
| Total score | | 10 |

## EXERCISE 2 ■ *Summary Activity*

Answers will vary for questions 13 through 16.

# Neonatology

## ■ Assignment

### Prerequisites:

- Complete Chapter 43, Neonatology, in *Mosby's Paramedic Textbook, Revised Third Edition.*
- Complete Chapter 43 in the workbook for *Mosby's Paramedic Textbook, Revised Third Edition.*
- Complete any skills or laboratory studies pertinent to this chapter.
- Read the "Getting Started" and "Orientation to Virtual Patient Encounters" sections in the *Virtual Patient Encounters Study Guide* (if this is the first lesson being attempted).

### Student assignment:

- Complete Lesson 38 in the *Virtual Patient Encounters Study Guide* after you have reviewed the topic in class.

## ■ Topic Review

### Objectives:

*On completion of this lesson, the student will be able to perform the following:*

- Anticipate resuscitation measures that may be needed for a prehospital delivery.
- Describe an appropriate sequence of events during neonatal resuscitation that could lead to a favorable outcome.

### Review the following topics with your students before they complete the lesson:

- At least 6% of neonates will need some type of resuscitation at birth. Paramedics must be prepared to deliver life-saving care to this unique patient group.
- A complicated birth has both antepartum and intrapartum risk factors. Antepartum factors include multiple gestation, maternal age younger than 16 or older than 35 years, history of perinatal death or injury, postterm gestation, drug use, toxemia, hypertension, and diabetes.
- Intrapartum factors related to fetal distress include premature labor, meconium-stained amniotic fluid, rupture of membranes more than 24 hours before delivery, narcotic use within 4 hours of delivery, abnormal presentation, prolonged labor, precipitous delivery, prolapsed cord, and bleeding.
- Four steps in assessment and management of the neonate are (1) prevent heat loss, (2) clear the airway, (3) provide tactile stimulation, and (3) further evaluate the neonate.
- All neonates are susceptible to hypothermia. At birth, the neonate should be dried and then covered (including the head) with warm blankets.

- Open the airway by placing the infant on his or her back or side with the head in a neutral position. A blanket may be placed under the infant's shoulders to maintain a neutral position. Suction the mouth and nose with a bulb syringe.

- If the infant needs further stimulation after drying, slap or flick the baby's feet and rub the infant's back.

- Further assessment should include evaluating respirations and continuing the examination if the respirations are normal, assessing the heart rate, and evaluating the infant's color. If acrocyanosis is noted, then hypoxemia is not indicated. If the infant's color is normal or improving, then assess the Apgar score.

- If the infant has inadequate respirations or heart rate, further resuscitation will be needed. This process may include reevaluation of the initial stabilization steps, ventilation, chest compressions, and, if no improvement is seen, administration of epinephrine or fluid.

# ■ Follow-Up

### *Assignment follow-up from previous class:*

- What problems, if any, did you have with your assignment?
- What questions do you have?

### *In-class activities and discussion questions:*

- Ask the class to describe the steps of resuscitation of a baby with thick meconium.
- Have the students draw a pyramid, and have them fill in the steps of neonatal resuscitation.

### *Other possible postcase activities:*

- Have students give a radio report detailing their care of the patient.
- Ask the class or a student group to evaluate the radio report.

### *Summary assessment:*

- Administer the quiz related to this lesson (Evolve resources, instructor's test bank).

# ■ STUDY GUIDE ANSWERS

### EXERCISE 1 ■ *Case 10: 25-year-old female—abdominal pain*

1. Based on the history that you have concerning this patient, explain whether you anticipate a high-risk delivery.

   **This delivery would be considered high risk. No prenatal care since early in the pregnancy was given; the baby is preterm; the mother has a history of prior fetal deaths; and the mother has signs and symptoms of toxemia with abdominal pain (might indicate abruptio).**

2. As the baby's head is delivered, you suction the airway. The shoulders then deliver quickly and you find yourself holding a floppy, blue baby. List your top four priorities at this time and the actions you will take to accomplish them.

| Priorities | Actions |
| --- | --- |
| Prevent heat loss. | Dry the baby and cover with warm blankets; ensure that the baby's head is covered; keep the ambulance warm; wrap the baby in commercial plastic wrap. |
| Clear the airway. | Position the baby on the back or side with the head in a neutral position; place a blanket under the baby's shoulders; suction the mouth and nose with a bulb syringe to clear the airway. |
| Provide tactile stimulation and begin breathing if needed. | Rub the baby's back, or flick the baby's feet. If no breathing is observed, then deliver breaths with a bag-mask. |
| Further evaluate the infant. | Check the pulse; if it is less than 100 bpm, begin ventilation; check for cyanosis (acrocyanosis is normal, central cyanosis is not). |

3. The baby is taking agonal gasps. Her heart rate is 50 beats per minute (bpm). She is very pale.
   a. What could account for her condition?

   **This delivery is considered high-risk, and a possibility exists of abruptio placenta because the mother's signs and symptoms suggest toxemia, and she had abdominal pain. The delivery is also early, and the mother has not had prenatal care for the last two trimesters of her pregnancy; therefore undetected problems may occur.**

   b. What are the immediate actions you need to take?

   **If you have already done the initial steps of resuscitation as previously described, and if the baby's heart rate does not improve rapidly after assisting her ventilation with a bag-mask, begin chest compressions.**

   c. If she does not respond favorably to your initial actions, what additional steps can you take?

   **If no improvement is seen, you will need to (as you prepare transport) attempt to establish vascular access quickly. A fluid bolus (normal saline or Ringer's lactate) of 10 mL/kg intravenously (IV) over 5 to 10 minutes might be administered, as well as epinephrine 0.01 to 0.03 mg/kg IV. If you are trained and authorized to do so, intubate the trachea. If any suspicion exists that the mother has used narcotics, naloxone can be given.**

4. Describe why intubation of this infant would be a high-risk procedure.

   **The infant is preterm, which increases the risk of vagal stimulation that can result in bradycardia. This intubation will be more difficult because of the size of the infant's airway and position of the epiglottis.**

# Pediatrics I

## ■ Assignment

### Prerequisites:

- Complete Chapter 44, Pediatrics, in *Mosby's Paramedic Textbook, Revised Third Edition.*
- Complete Chapter 44 in the workbook for *Mosby's Paramedic Textbook, Revised Third Edition.*
- Complete any skills or laboratory studies pertinent to this chapter.
- Read the "Getting Started" and "Orientation to Virtual Patient Encounters" sections in the *Virtual Patient Encounters Study Guide* (if this is the first lesson being attempted).

### Other relevant chapters:

In addition to Chapter 44, this lesson also draws content found in the following chapters:
- Chapter 3, Injury Prevention
- Chapter 7, General Principles of Pathophysiology
- Chapter 11, Techniques of Physical Examination
- Chapter 12, Patient Assessment
- Chapter 19, Airway Management and Ventilation
- Chapter 25, Spinal Trauma
- Chapter 38, Environmental Conditions

### Student assignment:

- Complete Lesson 39 in the *Virtual Patient Encounters Study Guide* after you have reviewed the topic in class.

## ■ Topic Review

### Objectives:

*On completion of this lesson, the student will be able to perform the following:*
- Identify the priorities of patient care based on an appropriate patient assessment.
- Predict potential injuries, based on the knowledge of mechanism of injury and relevant pathophysiologic characteristics.

### Review the following topics with your students before they complete the lesson:

- The drowning patient can present a complex clinical picture.
- Drowning is often complicated by traumatic injuries, environmental illness, or both.

- The drowning patient's signs and symptoms are ultimately the result of severe hypoxia. Untreated, the clinical picture of hypoxia can deteriorate quickly to death.
- Any drowning patient who requires any resuscitative measures, such as mouth-to-mouth resuscitation, even for a brief period, should be transported to the hospital for evaluation by a physician.
- Drowning events often involve children and are often difficult rescue situations that can be very emotional for the paramedic. Critical incident stress debriefing may be indicated if you or any of your crewmembers finds the call to be upsetting.
- Emergency medical services (EMS) providers can play an important role in drowning prevention activities.
- EMS providers can advocate for zoning that requires safety measures, such as fencing around pools. Educational programs can be taken to schools and community groups to educate children and their parents about pool safety.

# ■ Follow-Up

### Assignment follow-up from previous class:

- What problems, if any, did you have with your assignment?
- What questions do you have?

### In-class activities and discussion questions:

- Ask the class how they would manage hysterical friends or family members who are on the scene of a child drowning.
- Discuss factors that might cause large amounts of vomiting in a patient such as this one. Ask the students how they might minimize the risk of aspiration related to vomiting.

### Other possible postcase activities:

- Have students give a radio report detailing their care of the patient.
- Ask the class or a student group to evaluate the radio report.

### Summary assessment:

- Administer the quiz related to this lesson (Evolve resources, instructor's test bank).

# ■ STUDY GUIDE ANSWERS

### EXERCISE 1 ■ Case 7: 8-year-old male—submersion

1. What are some possible reasons why this child was submerged and lost consciousness?

   **Head injury, spinal cord injury, seizure, hypoglycemia, intoxication, inability to swim (hypoxia)**

2. Was the first-responder care appropriate? Explain your answer.

   **Although the first responder appeared to be holding manual in-line immobilization of the head, apparently, he was not opening the airway using the jaw-thrust maneuver or assessing respirations.**

3. If you had suggestions to change the care provided by the first responders, describe how you would address those concerns with them.

**Perhaps you might pull the first responder aside at a later time and nicely but directly suggest how he might change his care. For example, you might say. "Thanks for you help on that call—I'm glad you thought to get in-line immobilization right away—that was really important. I have one suggestion that you might try if you have a call like this again. While you're up at the head, you are in a perfect position to open the patient's airway and check for breathing. Here, let me show you what I mean."**

4. Explain why you selected the airway maneuvers and oxygen device and flow rate that you did.

**Because he had a history of diving and striking his head, minimizing movement of his spine was important. The jaw-thrust maneuver is appropriate for this patient. Initially, his airway was obstructed with secretions or vomit; thus suctioning the airway was necessary before inserting an oropharyngeal airway. While the intubation supplies are being set up, the patient is ventilated using a bag-mask. Intubating him for adequate ventilation and protecting his airway are necessary because he is at high risk for aspiration after drowning. The patient should be intubated, and, after intubation, continuous monitoring of tube placement should be performed.**

5. What factors will influence this patient's chance of survival?

**The most important determinant of survival from drowning is the duration of submersion and severity of hypoxia. Other factors include water temperature and cleanliness and age of the patient (younger patients have higher survival rates).**

6. Predict how the patient's condition might have changed if he had been rescued from the water 3 to 5 minutes later. Explain your answer.

**As the patient's hypoxia increased, his heart rhythm would have slowed until, finally, he would have developed pulseless electrical activity or became asystolic. Once in cardiac arrest, successful resuscitation becomes more difficult.**

7. Explain why the patient had the following signs or symptoms.

| Sign or Symptom | Pathophysiologic Basis for Sign or Symptom |
| --- | --- |
| Rhonchi | Two possible explanations for the rhonchi include the following: (1) In approximately 85% of drowning patients, water is aspirated into the airway, which causes the noise of rhonchi and contributes to hypoxia after rescue. (2) Patients who drown often swallow water and are at risk for vomiting and aspiration, which cause rhonchi. |
| Unconsciousness | The patient who drowns quickly develops hypoxia related to the lack of ambient oxygen. The brain is sensitive to even a momentary interruption of oxygen supply. Without it, consciousness deteriorates quickly. |

| Sign or Symptom | Pathophysiologic Basis for Sign or Symptom |
| --- | --- |
| Low oxygen saturation (SaO$_2$) | During drowning, hypoxia occurs by one of two mechanisms: (1) Water floods the airway, and no ambient oxygenated air is inhaled. (2) Severe laryngospasm occurs, and no air moves to the lower airways. With either cause, no oxygenated air reaches the alveoli. The cells quickly extract available oxygen dissolved in the blood and carried on the hemoglobin. The patient's oxygen saturation drops quickly, and acidosis develops. |

8. If you observed the following findings after you intubated the patient, explain what could cause them and what (if any) actions should be taken.

| Finding | Possible Causes | Actions |
| --- | --- | --- |
| SaO$_2$ is 72%. | Tube is displaced from trachea; airway is obstructed by secretions; patient has developed a pneumothorax; an equipment problem exists. | Reassess tube placement and correct if the tube is dislodged; suction the endotracheal tube to ensure that it is not blocked with secretions; assess for presence of breath sounds bilaterally and for presence of tension pneumothorax (decompress the chest if tension pneumothorax is present); check the equipment to ensure that oxygen supply is still adequate and that no problem exists with ventilation. If a ventilator is being used, switch to a bag-mask until problems can be corrected. |
| Breath sounds are heard over the right lung; breath sounds are absent over the left lung. | Probable intubation of right mainstem bronchus. | Deflate the cuff of the endotracheal tube and pull back slightly while listening to breathing sounds until bilateral breath sounds are audible. Reinflate the cuff, reassess, and secure the tube. |

| Finding | Possible Causes | Actions |
| --- | --- | --- |
| Initial finding is normal; 6 min after intubation you note (1) absence of breath sounds in the right lung, (2) subcutaneous emphysema in the anterior neck, (3) blood pressure (BP) 60 mm Hg by palpation, (4) $SaO_2$ is 70%. | **Probable tension pneumothorax.** | **Decrease volume of ventilation (ventilate with just enough volume to see chest rise). Decompress the chest with a 10- to 14-gauge catheter placed in the second intercostal space, midclavicular line. Reassess for hypoxia and signs of shock. Notify hospital to prepare for chest tube insertion.** |
| End-tidal $CO_2$ is 22. | **Normal end-tidal carbon dioxide is 35-45. Patient is receiving excessive minute volume during ventilation.** | **Adjust rate or volume (or both) of ventilation. Slow rate if too fast, and decrease volume if it is too great. Reassess end-tidal carbon dioxide to ensure it returns to a normal range.** |
| Esophageal detector device inflates in 6 seconds. | **Esophageal detector device should reinflate immediately if it is in the noncollapsible trachea.** | **Assess tube placement immediately by direct visualization and other clinical and device methods. If correct tube placement cannot be verified, then deflate the cuff, remove the tube, and ventilate the patient.** |

9. Assume you are unable to intubate this child. What are your options to manage his airway?

   **If intubation was not possible, and if a laryngeal mask airway of the appropriate pediatric size is available, it may be inserted to maintain the airway. If not, the child would be ventilated with an oropharyngeal airway in place using a bag-mask device. Great care should be taken to avoid overinflating the lungs because this child is at high risk of aspiration.**

10. What additional assessments and patient care measures would need to be taken if this event occurred on a day when the ambient temperature was 40° F (4° C)?

    **If this event were to occur on a cold day, measures to prevent further heat loss should be taken. The child's wet clothing would be removed, and he should be dried off and covered with a warm blanket. As soon as possible, he should be moved to the ambulance. If the determination is made that the patient is hypothermic, he would be ventilated with warmed, humidified oxygen, if available, and given warmed intravenous fluids.**

11. What actions would you take if the child were still submerged when you arrive?

   a. If the temperature were 86° F (30° C):

      **Rescuers trained in the proper techniques and who have sufficient safety devices to ensure that no other injuries occur during rescue should perform water rescue. The patient would need to be placed on a long spine board for removal from the water.**

   b. If the temperature were 10° F (–12° C):

      **If the ambient temperature is cold, persons who enter the water should wear specialized hypothermia suits. This requires additional training.**

12. Complete a patient care report (PCR) for this call. (Use one of the blank PCRs in the back of your study guide or one your instructor has given you.)

   **Each PCR will vary according to the treatment the student provided. Use the following guidelines to score the report. Some suggested significant information that should be noted is also included in italic print.**

   **PCR Evaluation Guidelines**

| Element | Suggested Completion | Maximum Score |
|---|---|---|
| **Chief complaint** | **Documented appropriately and completely** | **1** |
| | **Example:** | |
| | *Drowning* | |
| **Pertinent medical history** | **SAMPLE history and major medical history is documented accurately.** | **1** |
| | **Example:** | |
| | *S—Unresponsive, pulse present, diminished respirations, head laceration with minimal bleeding* | |
| | *A—Penicillin* | |
| | *M—Albuterol (Proventil) metered-dose inhaler* | |
| | *P—Asthma* | |
| | *L—Soda 30 minutes before* | |
| | *E—Patient's brother says he dove into the pool and did not come to surface.* | |
| **History of present illness** | **Events leading up to the illness or injury are clearly and concisely described in an appropriate sequence.** | **2** |
| | **Example:** | |
| | *Same as above and:* | |
| | *O—One minute before calling EMS* | |
| | *P—Diving into the pool* | |
| | *QRS—Unknown* | |
| | *T—One minute before calling EMS* | |

## PCR Evaluation Guidelines—*Continued*

| Element | Suggested Completion | Maximum Score |
|---|---|---|
| Physical examination | Appropriate physical examination that includes pertinent negatives is documented in a clear, concise manner using appropriate medical terminology. | 2 |
| | Example: | |
| | *Unresponsive, taking shallow breaths approximately 2 per minute; regular strong pulse present. Laceration 2" on anterior scalp with minimal bleeding, slight swelling around wound, breath sounds present bilaterally with rhonchi. Pupils dilated and react to light. Initially, fluid in airway cleared with suction; skin is pale and cool. No other injuries or abnormalities observed in focused assessment.* | |
| Sequence and readability | The narrative is written to clearly convey the sequence of the story and includes relevant details. | 1 |
| Vital signs | Initial vital signs and those obtained after each intervention and patient change are documented accurately and completely. | 1 |
| | NOTE: Vital signs documented should match those obtained in student log. | |
| Interventions | Complete documentation of interventions that includes sufficient details. | 2 |
| | *Airway management, oxygen administration, spinal immobilization. IV therapy includes volume and rate of administration. Patient positioning, warming, and other relevant interventions. Includes appropriate reassessments necessary to evaluate each intervention.* | |
| Total score | | 10 |

## EXERCISE 2 ■ *Summary Activity*

Answers will vary for questions 13 through 16.

# Pediatrics II

## ■ Assignment

### Prerequisites:

- Complete Chapter 44, Pediatrics, in *Mosby's Paramedic Textbook, Revised Third Edition.*
- Complete Chapter 44 in the workbook for *Mosby's Paramedic Textbook, Revised Third Edition.*
- Complete any skills or laboratory studies pertinent to this chapter.
- Read the "Getting Started" and "Orientation to Virtual Patient Encounters" sections in the *Virtual Patient Encounters Study Guide* (if this is the first lesson being attempted).

### Other relevant chapters:

In addition to Chapter 44, this lesson also draws content found in the following chapters:

- Chapter 3, Injury Prevention
- Chapter 4, Medical/Legal Issues
- Chapter 7, General Principles of Pathophysiology
- Chapter 8, Life Span Development
- Chapter 9, Therapeutic Communication
- Chapter 10, History Taking
- Chapter 11, Techniques of Physical Examination
- Chapter 12, Patient Assessment
- Chapter 16, Documentation
- Chapter 18, Venous Access and Medication Administration
- Chapter 19, Airway Management and Ventilation
- Chapter 29, Cardiology
- Chapter 46, Abuse and Neglect
- Chapter 47, Patients with Special Challenges

### Student assignment:

- Complete Lesson 40 in the *Virtual Patient Encounters Study Guide* after you have reviewed the topic in class.

# ■ Topic Review

## *Objectives:*

*On completion of this lesson, the student will be able to perform the following:*
- Perform a rapid assessment to determine the priorities of care in a critically ill child.
- Prioritize patient interventions to deliver the most effective care in a critically ill child.
- Use effective communication techniques to obtain an accurate history and to facilitate a therapeutic relationship with the child's parents.

### *Review the following topics with your students before they complete the lesson:*
- When you are dispatched to a call for an unresponsive infant, you need to anticipate what the possible causes might be so you can be prepared mentally and organize the right equipment to manage the patient as quickly and effectively as possible.
- The call can turn out to be a baby who is postictal, unconscious secondary to trauma, dehydrated, have drug toxicity, is septic, or is in cardiac arrest.
- Think about the special equipment and techniques you may need while you are en route to the call. Do you have a specialized pediatric bag? Do pediatric-specific protocols exist to which you can refer if needed? Do you know where the proper-sized bag-mask is located?
- You can often tell quickly whether a baby is in serious distress. Observe the baby as you approach. Is the baby alert? Is the baby moving, or is he or she floppy and without muscle tone? What is the baby's skin color? Do you see cyanosis or pallor, or is the baby pink?
- Open the airway. If the child is not breathing, first, give two breaths; then, assess the brachial pulse. If no pulse can be detected, then begin chest compressions.
- Attempt to gain intravenous access. If access is not possible, insert an intraosseous needle so you can administer fluids and drugs.
- If you are properly trained, and if your protocols permit, intubate the infant. Use the appropriate-sized tube, and confirm intubation often, using clinical methods and confirmation devices such as capnography. Be careful to avoid overinflating the lungs when delivering breaths.

# ■ Follow-Up

## *Assignment follow-up from previous class:*
- What problems, if any, did you have with your assignment?
- What questions do you have?

## *In-class activities and discussion questions:*
- What should you do if you are unable to intubate a baby?
- What should you consider when managing the airway of a 5-month-old infant based on your knowledge of the airway physiology at this age?

## *Other possible postcase activities:*
- Have students give a radio report detailing their care of the patient.
- Ask the class or a student group to evaluate the radio report.

*Summary assessment:*
- Administer the quiz related to this lesson (Evolve resources, instructor's test bank).

# ■ STUDY GUIDE ANSWERS

### EXERCISE 1 ■ *Case 13: 5-month-old male—unresponsive*

1. Name at least four situations that you should consider as you respond to this call, based on the dispatch information.

   **Sudden infant death syndrome (SIDS), seizure, sepsis, trauma**

2. What factors in this child's physical examination and medical history place him at increased risk for cardiac arrest?

   **This child's physical characteristics are consistent with Down syndrome: large, protruding tongue and low-set ears. Approximately 25% of children with Down syndrome have congenital heart defects. The cardiac arrest might be related to a preexisting heart problem.**

3. List at least six features of sudden infant death syndrome (SIDS). Indicate whether you observed any of these characteristics on this call.

| Characteristic | Observed on this Call? |
| --- | --- |
| Age <1 year (usually within the first 6 months) | Yes |
| Sudden death of seemingly healthy infant | Unknown history |
| Occurs during sleep | Yes |
| Usually between midnight and 6 AM | Yes |
| October through March (increased incidence) | Unknown |
| Minor illness before death | Unknown |
| Lividity | Unknown |
| Frothy, blood-tinged drainage from nose and mouth | Unknown cloudy fluid in mouth |
| Rigor mortis | No |
| Rumpled bed clothes or unusual position in bed | Unknown |

4. When you are on a noncardiac arrest call for an infant, what measures can you take to reduce the incidence of deaths related to SIDS?

   **If you are on a noncritical call and an infant is in the home, then mention to the parents the concept of placing the infant on his or her back (or on the side) to sleep. Educate the parents about the following actions that may decrease the risk of SIDS:**

   - **Avoid smoking around the infant.**
   - **Breast feed when possible.**
   - **Do not overheat the baby.**
   - **Attend well-baby check-ups at the physician.**

- **Maintain immunizations.**
- **Have the baby sleep on a firm mattress.**
- **Avoid putting the baby to sleep on or near beanbag cushions, waterbeds, fluffy blankets, sheepskins, pillows, or stuffed toys.**

5. What electrocardiographic (ECG) rhythm did you initially observe?

    **Ventricular fibrillation**

6. Explain why you did or did not choose to stop resuscitation of this infant on the scene.

    **You would continue resuscitation and transport this infant because ventricular fibrillation was present (not asystole) and because no clear evidence of rigor mortis was found.**

7. Explain why you selected the oxygen device and flow rate that you did.

    **Initially, an oropharyngeal airway was placed, and the patient was ventilated with a bag-mask device with 15 L/min oxygen delivery because he was in cardiac arrest. When possible, after good cardiopulmonary resuscitation and defibrillation, if properly trained rescuers are available, then the patient would be intubated.**

8. What additional physical findings were you looking for when you performed your focused history and physical examination?

    **You need to evaluate for airway obstruction, signs of lividity, signs of trauma, and other unusual physical features.**

9. Assume that each of the following drugs is needed in this situation. Calculate the proper amount of drug for this child who weighs 16 pounds.

    a. You are going to administer a second dose of adenosine 0.2 mg/kg. It is supplied in 6 mg per 2 ml vials. How many milliliters will you administer?

       **0.48 ml**

    b. You have to administer amiodarone 5 mg/kg. It is supplied in a 50 mg/ml vial. How many milliliters will you administer?

       **0.73 ml**

    c. You want to give naloxone 0.1 mg/kg. It is supplied in 0.4 mg/ml ampules. How many milliliters will you administer?

       **1.62 ml**

10. What communication techniques can you use if the baby's mother approaches you at the hospital to ask about his condition?

    a. Describe some general techniques you will use:

       **Try to sit down at eye level with the mother. Use the infant's name when you speak to the mother. Get a feel for what the mother thinks is happening. If you need to ask information, try to do so in a manner that does not appear to be an interrogation or in a manner that would appear to place blame on the mother.**

b. If she asks, "How's my baby?" What will be your reply?

**Explain that the baby was critically ill, had no pulse, and was not breathing. Tell the mother, in layman's terms, the things you did to try to resuscitate the baby, such as, "We breathed for him, gave him CPR to try and get some blood to his heart and brain, and gave him some drugs to try and restart his heart and breathing." Honestly explain that the things you did for her baby did not help. Let the mother know that a physician and nursing staff are with her baby still trying to help him.**

11. Complete a patient care report (PCR) for this call. (Use one of the PCRs in the back of your study guide or one your instructor has given you.)

**Each PCR will vary according to the treatment the student provided. Use the following guidelines to score the report. Some suggested significant information that should be noted is also included in italic print.**

### PCR Evaluation Guidelines

| Element | Suggested Completion | Maximum Score |
|---|---|---|
| **Chief complaint** | **Documented appropriately and completely** | 1 |
| **Pertinent medical history** | **SAMPLE history and major medical history is documented accurately.** | 1 |
| | **Example:** | |
| | *S—Unresponsive, apneic, pulseless* | |
| | *A—Unknown* | |
| | *M—Unknown* | |
| | *P—Unknown; large tongue, low-set ears, consistent with Down syndrome* | |
| | *L—Unknown* | |
| | *E—Mother found baby unresponsive when she went in to check on him this morning.* | |
| **History of present illness** | **Events leading up to the illness or injury are clearly and concisely described in an appropriate sequence.** | 2 |
| | **Example:** | |
| | *Unknown, except as above. Found outside the home in mother's arms.* | |
| **Physical examination** | **Appropriate physical examination that includes pertinent negatives is documented in a clear, concise manner using appropriate medical terminology.** | 2 |
| | **Example:** | |
| | *Unresponsive, apneic, pulseless infant. Pupils dilated and nonreactive. Cyanotic; no chest excursion, no breath sounds. Small amount of cloudy fluid in nose and mouth—suctioned. Blood glucose 50 mg/dl.* | |

**PCR Evaluation Guidelines**—*Continued*

| Element | Suggested Completion | Maximum Score |
|---|---|---|
| Sequence and readability | The narrative is written to clearly convey the sequence of the story and includes relevant details. | 1 |
| Vital signs | Initial vital signs and those obtained after each intervention and patient change are documented accurately and completely. | 1 |
| | NOTE: Vital signs documented should match those obtained in student log. | |
| Interventions | Complete documentation of interventions that includes sufficient details. | 2 |
| | *Oxygen administration, drugs with appropriate route, dose, and rate of administration. IV therapy includes volume and rate of administration. Defibrillation energy levels, CPR, patient positioning, and other relevant interventions. Includes appropriate reassessments necessary to evaluate each intervention.* | |
| Total score | | 10 |

## EXERCISE 2 ■ *Summary Activity*

Answers will vary for questions 12 through 15.

# Geriatrics

## ▉ Assignment

### Prerequisites:

- Complete Chapter 45, Geriatrics, in *Mosby's Paramedic Textbook, Revised Third Edition*.
- Complete Chapter 45 in the workbook for *Mosby's Paramedic Textbook, Revised Third Edition*.
- Complete any skills or laboratory studies pertinent to this chapter.
- Read the "Getting Started" and "Orientation to Virtual Patient Encounters" sections in the *Virtual Patient Encounters Study Guide* (if this is the first lesson being attempted).

### Student assignment:

- Complete Lesson 41 in the *Virtual Patient Encounters Study Guide* after you have reviewed the topic in class.

## ▉ Topic Review

### Objectives:

*On completion of this lesson, the student will be able to perform the following:*

- Recognize physical and psychosocial influences that aging may have on this patient.
- Distinguish the characteristics between normal age-related changes and pathologic changes in this patient.

### Review the following topics with your students before they complete the lesson:

- As the number of older adults grows in this country, the number of ambulance transports will rise proportionately. Paramedics must recognize how age-related changes affect delivery of emergency care.
- All body systems are affected by aging. Some of these changes may require alterations in patient assessment and management.
- The respiratory system loses elasticity and some of its protective functions with increasing age. In the seventh decade, the vital capacity decreases by approximately 50%, and partial pressure of arterial oxygen is 70 mm Hg. Carbon dioxide levels do not change with normal aging.
- The incidence of arteriosclerotic heart disease increases with age. The ability of the heart to respond to stressors also declines. By 80 years of age, cardiac output has decreased 30%. Physiologic changes in the cardiac electrical system predispose the aging patient to dysrhythmias.
- Renal blood flow declines 50% between the ages of 30 and 80 years. This decrease makes the patient more susceptible to renal failure related to trauma, infection, obstruction, or vascular occlusion. Electrolyte disturbances and altered response to drug therapy may result from renal function decline.

**200**

- Changes in the nervous system can alter motor or position sense and cause delays in reaction time and motor response. Vision and hearing may also diminish as patients age.
- Muscles shrink and calcify, and intervertebral disks thin as the body ages. Osteoporosis is common, especially in older women. Falls are common in the older adult and result in significant injuries and high mortality.
- Other age-related changes include decreasing ability to maintain homeostasis, maintain body temperature, and fight infection. Additionally, the incidence of malnutrition is increased in this age group.
- Assessment and care of the older adult can be challenging because of sensory changes, multiple chronic disease processes, altered response to injury or illness, altered response to pain, and fear of hospitalization and social challenges in this age-group.

## ■ Follow-Up

### Assignment follow-up from previous class:

- What problems, if any, did you have with your assignment?
- What questions do you have?

### In-class activities and discussion questions:

- Obtain a shirt or a pair of slacks that is old and has worn, stretched-out elastic. Ask the students to relate the changes in the elastic to the changes in the vascular system of the older adult.
- Ask the class to gather health information on one relative who is over 65 years of age. What illness does this person have? What medications does the person take? How does the person function and cope with his or her illnesses?

### Summary assessment:

- Administer the quiz related to this lesson (Evolve resources, instructor's test bank).

## ■ STUDY GUIDE ANSWERS

### EXERCISE 1 ■ Case 14: 65-year-old male—difficulty breathing

1. List at least two age-related changes observed in this patient as you watched the initial video clip.

   **The patient has gray hair, and his skin is wrinkled. His posture seems somewhat kyphotic.**

2. How might potential age-related changes in the following body systems affect your care?

| Action to Be Performed | Body System | Effect on Assessment or Patient Care? |
|---|---|---|
| Blood pressure assessment | Cardiovascular | **You would anticipate his blood pressure is slightly higher than normal, unless he is taking medicine to control it.** |

| Action to Be Performed | Body System | Effect on Assessment or Patient Care? |
|---|---|---|
| Administration of sublingual tablets | Gastrointestinal tract | **Because older adults tend to have reduced production of saliva, sublingual tablets may take longer to dissolve and be absorbed.** |
| Breath sound assessment | Respiratory system | **The patient may be unable to take really deep breaths if needed during this assessment.** |
| Establishing vascular access | Integumentary and vascular systems | **You may need to apply less tourniquet pressure when establishing intravenous (IV) access because veins are more fragile. Veins may appear more tortuous and not travel straight. Select a tape or IV-securing adhesive dressing that is not so aggressive that it will pull off skin when removed.** |

3. Why might this patient be noncompliant with his prescription medications?

   **Older adults may be noncompliant with medications for many reasons, including: the inability to pay for expensive medicines while on a fixed income; inability to leave the house to get the prescription; the patient may have a history of dementia or Alzheimer's disease, making the patient too confused to take medicines properly; the patient may be unable to read the instructions for administration properly if vision is impaired; or the patient may be unable to remove the safety cap to open his medicines because of arthritis or decreased strength in the hands.**

4. State whether each of the following physical findings would be an expected, age-related change. If each finding is expected, then explain the physiologic alteration that causes the change; if it is not, then state at least one cause of the finding.

| Function | Age-Related? | Explanation |
|---|---|---|
| Partial pressure of arterial oxygen ($PaO_2$)—70 torr | **Yes** | **The $PaO_2$ declines with age. On average, it would be in this range at 70 years of age.** |
| Carbon dioxide ($CO_2$)—55 torr | **No** | **If the $CO_2$ is elevated, then it indicates a disease process or impaired ventilation; $CO_2$ does not decline as a normal change in aging.** |
| Blood pressure—140/90 mm Hg | **Yes** | **As the walls of the blood vessels stiffen with age, blood pressure increases.** |

5. What factor did you observe in your scene size-up that may mean that your assessment of this patient's dyspnea could be complicated?

**This patient is using home oxygen, which means that he has a preexisting pulmonary condition that causes hypoxia. Unless the patient is well educated, he may not know what his normal oxygen saturation level is. Additionally, interpreting his level of distress may be difficult if you are unfamiliar with his baseline status.**

6. What should you look for in this patient's environment that would indicate he is having difficulty in maintaining normal activities of daily living?

**Assess the surroundings for cleanliness and any evidence that he has been incontinent of urine or feces (because he cannot ambulate). He appears to be thin. Check the kitchen for evidence of food or ask the patient how he gets his meals (he may have a service bring them in for him). Determine if the house temperature is safe (some older adults are reluctant to heat or cool their properly homes because they cannot afford it).**

7. What techniques of effective communication did you observe on this call?

**The paramedics knocked first and entered. Then, they introduced themselves and crouched down to the patient's eye level. They did not use demeaning terms and addressed the patient by his name. They told him what they were going to do before they did anything (put the dog in another room).**

# Abuse and Neglect

## ◼ Assignment

### Prerequisites:

- Complete Chapter 46, Abuse and Neglect, in *Mosby's Paramedic Textbook, Revised Third Edition*.
- Complete Chapter 46 in the workbook for *Mosby's Paramedic Textbook, Revised Third Edition*.
- Complete any skills or laboratory studies pertinent to this chapter.
- Read the "Getting Started" and "Orientation to Virtual Patient Encounters" sections in the *Virtual Patient Encounters Study Guide* (if this is the first lesson being attempted).

### Other relevant chapters:

In addition to Chapter 46, this lesson also draws content found in the following chapters:
- Chapter 4, Medical/Legal Issues
- Chapter 7, General Principles of Pathophysiology
- Chapter 9, Therapeutic Communication
- Chapter 11, Techniques of Physical Examination
- Chapter 12, Patient Assessment
- Chapter 16, Documentation
- Chapter 17, Pharmacology
- Chapter 22, Soft Tissue Trauma
- Chapter 23, Burns
- Chapter 24, Head and Facial Trauma
- Chapter 25, Spinal Trauma
- Chapter 36, Toxicology
- Chapter 52, Crime Scene Awareness

### Student assignment:

- Complete Lesson 42 in the *Virtual Patient Encounters Study Guide* after you have reviewed the topic in class.

## ◼ Topic Review

### Objectives:

*On completion of this lesson, the student will be able to perform the following:*
- Outline care for the physical and psychologic needs of a patient who has been subjected to physical, sexual, or emotional abuse.

204

- Discuss how to integrate principles of crime scene preservation during the assessment and management of a patient who has been subjected to physical, sexual, or emotional abuse.
- Document the call appropriately.

### *Review the following topics with your students before they complete the lesson:*

- As with every call, the first priority when you respond to an assault is to ensure that the scene is safe. Never assume that, just because you have been told by law enforcement that the scene is secure, that it is entirely safe. Be vigilant during the entire call in case the situation deteriorates and the scene becomes unsafe.
- Once scene safety is established, assess for and manage life threats. After the life threats have been addressed, consider the emotional needs of the patient. The injuries are often resolved long before the emotional effects of the call are controlled. In the case of reported sexual assault, physical examination of the patient's genitalia is unnecessary unless any bleeding is noted or reported.
- Your primary goal to support these patients' emotional needs is to ensure their safety. Make statements about safety precautions you are taking, and reassure the patients.
- It is also important to accept the patients' story without undue questions that do not relate directly to your patient care. Determining the exact facts that surround the incident will be the job of the police, not emergency medical services (EMS) personnel.
- Take measures to preserve the crime scene if the patient is at the location where the incident occurred. Do not move objects or walk through liquids or blood unless absolutely needed for patient care.
- Try not to disturb any evidence. If the patient's clothing or belongings are removed, place them in an appropriate container that will not destroy evidence, and give the container to the police. The evidence should remain with you until you and the police have documented that you have given it to them.
- Documentation of these situations should be performed with special care and should include direct quotes (if you remember them exactly) documented in quotation marks. Include statements about the exact size and location of injuries and the details regarding any evidence that you have turned over to law enforcement.

## ■ Follow-Up

### *Assignment follow-up from previous class:*

- What problems, if any, did you have with your assignment?
- What questions do you have?

### *In-class activities and discussion questions:*

- Discuss the role and benefit of nurses who specialize in the care of the rape patient.

### *Other possible postcase activities:*

- Have students give a radio report detailing their care of the patient.
- Ask the class or a student group to evaluate the radio report.

### *Summary assessment:*

- Administer the quiz related to this lesson (Evolve resources, instructor's test bank).

# ■ STUDY GUIDE ANSWERS

### EXERCISE 1 ■ *Case 9: 22-year-old female—assault*

1. Based on the initial information you received from dispatch and your initial assessment, list at least four injuries or illnesses that you may encounter on this call.

   **Burns, soft-tissue trauma, overdose or intoxication, sexual assault, emotional trauma**

2. As you enter the room to assess and manage the patient, what are your priorities?

   **After establishing that the scene is safe, perform an initial assessment to determine the presence of life threats related to airway, breathing, or circulation. Manage life threats identified in the initial assessment.**

3. Describe why you believe the patient should or should not have spinal immobilization (spinal motion restriction).

   **The exact mechanism of injury to the jaw is unknown. However, if severe trauma to the jaw is evident, then the neck may have been injured. If your protocols permit, use spinal immobilization rule out criteria on the patient to assess the need for immobilization. First, ensure that the patient is reliable (not incompetent), ask if she has spine pain. Palpate over each spinous process to assess for pain. Then, evaluate upper and lower extremity motor and sensory function. If any aspect of the examination is abnormal, the patient should be immobilized.**

4. Why should you exercise extreme caution if you elect to administer pain medicine to this patient?

   **The patient was reportedly given drugs; however, you have no information related to the type of drugs, how much, or the route that was used. Narcotic analgesics can potentiate the hypotensive and respiratory depressive effects of illicit drugs. Administer analgesia with caution, and prepare to manage any side effects.**

5. Describe the detailed assessment you would perform on this patient's jaw.

   **Inspect for asymmetry, swelling, or wounds over the lower facial bones. If possible, and if it does not cause the patient undue pain, ask the patient to open her mouth. If she can open it, then assess for malocclusion of the teeth, for blood or loose teeth in the mouth that have the potential to obstruct the airway, and for numbness over the chin. Ask the patient if her teeth "feel right" when her mouth is closed.**

6. Describe signs or symptoms that would lead you to suspect that this patient has an inhalation injury.

   **Signs and symptoms that indicate the potential for inhalation injury are the burns of the face, nose, and mouth. However, the mechanism of injury, which was scalding water, is not consistent with a risk of inhalation injury.**

7. Explain your rationale for the genital examination you should perform on this patient.

   **No genital examination would be appropriate for this patient. No report of bleeding or severe injury in this area has been made. Any attempt to examine her perineum may increase her level of emotional distress and has the potential to destroy evidence.**

8. List the specific injury you suspect and at least one possible complication related to the injuries you observed in the patient on this call.

| Sign or Symptom | Specific Injury Suspected | Possible Complications |
|---|---|---|
| Burns around nose or mouth | Partial-thickness burn | Pain, infection, scarring (if infection occurs) |
| Severe pain of the jaw | Fractured mandible | Airway compromise, pain |

9. For each drug that you administered in this case, describe at least two effects it had and the reason for these effects.

| Drug | Effect | Explanation |
|---|---|---|
| Morphine | Decreased pain | Blocks central pain receptors. |
| | Decreased oxygen saturation, decreased depth of respiration | Side effects of narcotic may be enhanced by other illicit drugs given to the patient. |
| Fentanyl | Decreased pain | Blocks central pain receptors. |
| | Decreased oxygen saturation, decreased depth of respiration | Side effects of narcotic may be enhanced by other illicit drugs given to the patient. |

10. Graph the heart rate and oxygen saturation ($SaO_2$) that you obtained (consult your log). Connect the data points so that each vital sign forms a line (see example on page 258 of the Study Guide). Use blue ink for the heart rate and red ink for $SaO_2$.
    - **Each graph will be individual and based on the interventions that the student selected.**
    - **Ideally the heart rate should go down as the patient's pain is relieved.**

11. Referring to your own graph, answer the following questions:
    a. What trends do you observe?
    b. How did your interventions relate to the trends you observe?
    c. If the trend reversed at any point, then how can you explain that variation?
    **Answers will vary to these questions.**

12. Should you ask the police officer to leave so you can protect the patient's rights as granted by the Health Insurance Portability and Accountability Act (HIPAA) of 1996? Explain your answer.
    **No. Allow the police office to remain with the patient. Patients who have been assaulted often feel safer in the presence of a caregiver of the same sex. Ask the patient for her wishes in this regard. If you are unsure, then have the officer remain with her until you arrive at the hospital if possible.**

13. Complete a patient care report (PCR) for this call. (Use one of the blank PCRs in the back of your study guide or one your instructor has given you.)

**Each PCR will vary according to the treatment the student provided. Use the following guidelines to score the report. Some suggested significant information that should be noted is also included in italic print.**

## PCR Evaluation Guidelines

| Element | Suggested Completion | Maximum Score |
|---|---|---|
| Chief complaint | Documented appropriately and completely<br>Example:<br>*Assault* | 1 |
| Pertinent medical history | SAMPLE history and major medical history is documented accurately.<br>Example:<br>*S—Blunt trauma to the face; deformed jaw, burns to the face, neck, and upper chest. Lacerations to the right arm.*<br>*A—Denies*<br>*M—Denies*<br>*P—Denies*<br>*L—Drank water 3 hours ago.*<br>*E—Held captive and assaulted (emotionally, sexually, physically).* | 1 |
| History of present illness | Events leading up to the illness or injury are clearly and concisely described in an appropriate sequence.<br>Example:<br>*Same as above and:*<br>*O—Incident began last night.*<br>*P—Movement of face, jaw, neck, and arms creates increased pain.*<br>*Q—Pain is severe and sharp.*<br>*R—Upper body and face; no visible physical trauma or bleeding to genitalia.*<br>*S—9/10*<br>*T—She estimates that the sexual assault occurred 4 hours before the call to EMS; trauma to the jaw and arms—approximately 2 hours before the call; she was burned with scalding water approximately 30 minutes ago.* | 2 |

## PCR Evaluation Guidelines—*Continued*

| Element | Suggested Completion | Maximum Score |
|---|---|---|
| Physical examination | Appropriate physical examination that includes pertinent negatives is documented in a clear, concise manner using appropriate medical terminology.<br><br>**Example:**<br><br>*Alert and oriented × 3. Respirations shallow, rapid. Breath sounds clear and equal bilaterally. Pulse is 116 breaths/min, regular and strong. Jaw is painful, deformed, and swollen. Small blisters on end of nose and around mouth. Swollen lips. Partial thickness burns over face and neck (4.5%). Face and neck extremely tender. Partial-thickness burns of upper chest. Two puncture wounds on inner aspect of right arm. Two lacerations (approximately 2 inches each) on inner aspect of right arm. Skin pink, warm, and dry.* | 2 |
| Sequence and readability | The narrative is written to clearly convey the sequence of the story and includes relevant details. | 1 |
| Vital signs | Initial vital signs and those obtained after each intervention and patient change are documented accurately and completely.<br><br>**NOTE:** Vital signs documented should match those obtained in student log. | 1 |
| Interventions | Complete documentation of interventions that includes sufficient details.<br><br>*Oxygen administration, measures to clear and maintain airway; drugs with appropriate route, dose. and rate of administration. IV therapy includes volume and rate of administration. Patient positioning and other relevant interventions. Includes appropriate reassessments necessary to evaluate each intervention.* | 2 |
| Total score | | 10 |

## EXERCISE 2 ■ *Summary Activity*

Answers will vary for questions 14 through 17.

# Patients with Special Challenges

## ■ Assignment

### Prerequisites:

- Complete Chapter 47, Patients with Special Challenges, in *Mosby's Paramedic Textbook, Revised Third Edition*.
- Complete Chapter 47 in the workbook for *Mosby's Paramedic Textbook, Revised Third Edition*.
- Complete any skills or laboratory studies pertinent to this chapter.
- Read the "Getting Started" and "Orientation to Virtual Patient Encounters" sections in the *Virtual Patient Encounters Study Guide* (if this is the first lesson being attempted).

### Student assignment:

- Complete Lesson 43 in the *Virtual Patient Encounters Study Guide* after you have reviewed the topic in class.

## ■ Topic Review

### Objectives:

*On completion of this lesson, the student will be able to perform the following:*

- Describe alterations in normal physiologic function related to selected patients with special challenges.
- Recognize physical attributes consistent with diseases or conditions that create special challenges.
- Outline the modifications in prehospital patient management that may be necessary when dealing with selected patients with special challenges.

### Review the following topics with your students before they complete the lesson:

- Paramedics must have a fundamental understanding of patients with unique physical, emotional, pathologic, or financial situations so they can provide appropriate care despite the significant challenges these patients may pose.
- A chromosomal defect is responsible for Down syndrome. Patients who have Down syndrome have variable mental disabilities. A significant number of persons with Down syndrome have heart defects and other illnesses.
- Cerebral palsy is a nonprogressive disorder of movement and posture resulting from damage to the infant's brain in utero, during birth, or in early infancy.
- The three types of cerebral palsy are (1) spastic paralysis, (2) athetosis, and (3) ataxia. Approximately 60% of persons with cerebral palsy have mental retardation.

- Obese patients are 30% above their ideal body weight. Obesity increases the risk of heart disease, diabetes, and other illnesses.
- Specialized equipment and extra assistance is usually necessary when caring for obese patients to assess and move them safely without injury to the patient or emergency medical services (EMS) crew.
- Obese patients are often self-conscious about their weight. EMS crews should treat these patients with respect and take measures to protect their privacy and dignity.

## ■ Follow-Up

### Assignment follow-up from previous class:

- What problems, if any, did you have with your assignment?
- What questions do you have?

### In-class activities and discussion questions:

- Ask students to describe the type of patients with special needs who they find to be most challenging to care for. Explore the students' reasons and see if the other students have some strategies to assist them.

### Summary assessment:

- Administer the quiz related to this lesson (Evolve resources, instructor's test bank).

## ■ STUDY GUIDE ANSWERS

### EXERCISE 1 ■ Case 2: 56-year-old female—fell

1. Assuming that this patient is 5 foot 2 inches and weighs 440 pounds, answer the following questions.

    a. Calculate this patient's body mass index (BMI). (Use the information in Box 2-6 on page 27 of your textbook.)

    **Step one: Multiply the weight in pounds times 0.45 (440 × 0.45 = 198).**

    **Step two: Multiply the height in inches (62) times 0.025 (62 × 0.025 = 1.55); square your previous answer (1.55 × 1.55 = 2.4025)**

    **Step three: Divide the answer in step one by the answer in step two (198 ÷ 2.4025 = 82.41)**

    b. In which category does this BMI place her?
    
    i. Healthful
    
    ii. Moderately overweight
    
    iii. Severely overweight

    **This patient's BMI is 82. This value puts her in the severely overweight category.**

2. List three possible causes for this patient's obesity.

    **Caloric intake exceeds calories burned, low basal metabolic rate, genetic predisposition for obesity.**

3. What medical conditions should you anticipate in a morbidly obese patient?

   **Bariatric patients are at high risk for hypertension, stroke, heart disease, diabetes, some cancers, and osteoporosis.**

4. What modifications may need to be made when performing the physical examination of this patient?

   **A large blood pressure cuff will be needed, electrocardiogram (ECG) leads should be placed in areas with the least fat, and you may need assistance to position the patient to auscultate breath sounds.**

## EXERCISE 2 ■ *Case 3: 7-year-old female—seizure*

5. This child's parent indicates that the patient has a history of cerebral palsy. What causes cerebral palsy?

   **Cerebral palsy is caused by damage to the fetal brain in late pregnancy, during birth, or in infancy or early childhood. The most common cause is abnormal fetal brain development. Other causes include fetal hypoxia, birth trauma, maternal infection, excessive bilirubin, encephalitis, meningitis, and head injury.**

6. Distinguish the physical manifestations among the three types of cerebral palsy.

| Spastic Paralysis | Athetosis | Ataxia |
|---|---|---|
| Stiffness and contraction of muscle groups. Diplegia affects all four limbs (legs more than arms); hemiplegia affects one side; quadriplegia affects all four limbs. | Involuntary writhing movements | Loss of coordination and balance |

7. Do all patients with cerebral palsy have severe mental retardation? Explain your answer.

   **Approximately 60% of persons with cerebral palsy have mental retardation. Of the other 40%, some are highly intelligent.**

8. What are the considerations for prehospital care of this patient?

   **Patients with spastic cerebral palsy may be positioned in specialized chairs with padding to support and control severe spasticity. A large amount of padding may be needed to position the patient comfortably on the ambulance stretcher. Communication may be difficult if the patient has severe mental retardation. If possible, have a parent or caregiver assist you.**

## EXERCISE 3 ■ *Case 13: 5-month-old male—unresponsive*

9. Your initial observation of this child indicates physical characteristics of Down syndrome. List other physical characteristics that indicate Down syndrome.

   **Upward sloping eyes, folds of skin on nose that cover medial aspects of eyes, large tongue, small face, flattened back of head, short, broad hands**

10. What physical problems are common in patients with Down syndrome?

    **Approximately 25% have congenital heart defects. Many people with Down syndrome have intestinal problems, hearing defects, or other illnesses such as leukemia.**

11. If you encounter an older patient with Down syndrome, what modifications might you need to make during your initial assessment to accommodate this patient's condition?

    **You may need to allow extra time to obtain the history and perform the physical examination.**

# Acute Interventions for the Home Health Care Patient

## ■ Assignment

### Prerequisites:

- Complete Chapter 48, Acute Interventions for the Home Health Care Patient, in *Mosby's Paramedic Textbook, Revised Third Edition*.
- Complete Chapter 48 in the workbook for *Mosby's Paramedic Textbook, Revised Third Edition*.
- Complete any skills or laboratory studies pertinent to this chapter.
- Read the "Getting Started" and "Orientation to Virtual Patient Encounters" sections in the *Virtual Patient Encounters Study Guide* (if this is the first lesson being attempted).

### Student assignment:

- Complete Lesson 44 in the *Virtual Patient Encounters Study Guide* after you have reviewed the topic in class.

## ■ Topic Review

### Objectives:

*On completion of this lesson, the student will be able to perform the following:*

- Predict oxygen equipment problems that may be encountered by a home care patient.
- Identify resources for the home care patient who has an oxygen equipment problem.

### Review the following topics with your students before they complete the lesson:

- Acute home health care emergencies may be related to equipment failure or improper operation of the equipment; deterioration in the patient's condition may also cause home health care emergencies.
- When called to evaluate a patient with complex home health interventions, the paramedic should perform a standard initial assessment and then determine a course of action based on the patient assessment and knowledge of specific equipment-related considerations.
- Oxygen therapy in the home may be supplied by compressed gas, liquid oxygen, or an oxygen concentrator.
- Home oxygen may be administered by nasal cannula, oxygen masks, tracheostomy collars, or ventilators.
- Some patients may need continuous positive-pressure delivery into the pulmonary system. This pressure may be delivered by continuous positive airway pressure (CPAP) or biphasic positive airway pressure (BiPAP) devices.

- Home ventilators may be volume, pressure, or negative-pressure ventilators. Ventilator settings include oxygen, volume, rate, inspiratory flow, sensitivity, and sigh rate.
- When assessing patients on home oxygen therapy, evaluate their work of breathing, tidal volume, peak flow, and breath sounds.
- Observe for signs of hypoxia such as confusion, cyanosis, dyspnea, headache, hypertension, hyperventilation, restlessness, and tachycardia.
- Interventions should be aimed at improving airway patency, ventilation, and oxygenation.

# ■ Follow-Up

### *Assignment follow-up from previous class:*

- What problems, if any, did you have with your assignment?
- What questions do you have?

### *In-class activities and discussion questions:*

- Borrow an oxygen concentrator to show your class.
- Ask the students to review the DOPE mnemonic (**d**isplaced tube, **o**bstruction, **p**neumothorax, or **e**quipment problem) to troubleshoot for a patient who is on a home ventilator and having problems.

### *Summary assessment:*

- Administer the quiz related to this lesson (Evolve resources, instructor's test bank).

# ■ STUDY GUIDE ANSWERS

### EXERCISE 1 ■ *Case 14: 65-year-old male—difficulty breathing*

1. When you see that the patient is on home oxygen, how does this circumstance contribute to your initial impression of the patient's condition?

   **When the patient has home oxygen, the therapy has likely been prescribed to treat a chronic pulmonary condition. The patient's baseline oxygenation and oxygen saturation is often low; therefore determining what is normal would be important for the patient.**

2. What type of oxygen supply does this patient have? What are the advantages and disadvantages of this type of supply as compared with an oxygen concentrator?

| | Patient's Oxygen | Other |
|---|---|---|
| Type | **Compressed gas** | Oxygen concentrator |
| Advantages | **Can run without electricity; is portable** | **Does not require constant resupply of oxygen** |
| Disadvantages | **Must have frequent resupply; poses potential hazard in the presence of fire** | **Must have constant electricity source to deliver oxygen** |

3. If this patient's condition were to improve immediately when you removed his nasal cannula and placed him on your tank and your equipment, what specific equipment problems should you suspect?

**If his condition improves immediately, then his home oxygen delivery system has a problem. If he is using compressed gas, check the regulator to ensure it is set on the proper liter flow, check the amount of gas in the bottle to ensure it is not empty, and check the tubing for kinks or leaks that may impair flow. If he is using an oxygen concentrator, check the power source and connections on the machine, and check the tubing as you would for a compressed gas tank.**

4. What will you do if:

a. This patient calls and says that his oxygen tank will run out in 2 hours:

**Assess the patient for the presence of an acute emergency situation. Have him contact his supplier to determine when an emergency supply is available. If it will be delayed greater than the time remaining, have him contact his personal physician to determine whether the patient is stable enough to be off oxygen for this period. Contact medical direction for advice. You may have to transport if the patient becomes hypoxic off of oxygen and no other option is available.**

b. This patient is on an oxygen concentrator, and the power is out in his home:

**Evaluate the patient for the presence of an acute emergency. Patients who are on oxygen concentrators should have a back-up compressed gas supply. Assist the patient to connect to the compressed gas supply, and determine if you can help the patient find transportation to a location with a power source (family or friend's home or emergency shelter).**

c. This patient is on an oxygen concentrator, and the power is out in your entire district:

**Perform the same activities as described in point 4b, and determine if aid is available through the Red Cross or another community agency to find temporary lodging for this patient.**

d. This patient comes up to your station and asks you to fill his oxygen tank because his will be empty tomorrow:

**Administration and dispensing of oxygen is controlled the same as prescription medicines. Generally, emergency medical services agencies are not authorized to dispense oxygen to individuals. Assist the patient to contact his or her provider of oxygen to obtain a refill.**

# Ambulance Operations

## ■ Assignment

### Prerequisites:

- Complete Chapter 49, Ambulance Operations, in *Mosby's Paramedic Textbook, Revised Third Edition*.
- Complete Chapter 49 in the workbook for *Mosby's Paramedic Textbook, Revised Third Edition*.
- Complete any skills or laboratory studies pertinent to this chapter.
- Read the "Getting Started" and "Orientation to Virtual Patient Encounters" sections in the *Virtual Patient Encounters Study Guide* (if this is the first lesson being attempted).

### Student assignment:

- Complete Lesson 45 in the *Virtual Patient Encounters Study Guide* after you have reviewed the topic in class.

## ■ Topic Review

### Objectives:

*On completion of this lesson, the student will be able to perform the following:*
- Relate the need for specialty resources to this case.
- Describe appropriate helicopter safety procedures as they relate to this case.

### Review the following topics with your students before they complete the lesson:

- Safe ambulance operation is a critical aspect of the role of the paramedic to protect the public, the community, and the emergency medical services (EMS) crew.
- Safe operations include using safety restraints, being alert to changes in weather conditions, exercising caution when using audible and visual warning devices, driving within the speed limit except as allowed by law, maintaining a safe following distance, and driving with due regard for the safety of others.
- Lights and sirens should be used judiciously and with caution. Do not use one without the other. Weigh the risks of using lights and sirens against the benefits for your patient. Follow local protocols. Most state laws will only permit ambulance crews to exceed the posted speed limit when lights and sirens are used.
- Over one-half of collisions occur in intersections. Stop at all controlled intersections when you do not have the right of way. Make eye contact with other drivers. Change your siren tone to yelp, or use your air horn to notify other drivers of your presence. Use traffic signal preempting devices if they are available.

**217**

- If other emergency responders are on the scene, position the ambulance 100 feet past the incident. Use emergency lighting when your ambulance blocks traffic. Set the parking brake. Use a guide when backing up the ambulance. Wear reflective gear when working on the roadway.

- Aeromedical transport protocols vary widely by EMS system. Follow your local guidelines. Generally, air medical transport in an emergency is used when the time for ground transport might allow the patient's situation to deteriorate, or if local conditions would delay advanced life support response, or if specialized equipment or personnel are needed to transport a patient safely.

- On-scene providers should select a landing zone that is at least 100 × 100 feet. It should be free of overhead obstructions, high grass, or uneven terrain. Rescuers in the vicinity of the landing zone should wear protective eyewear and cover the patient's face while the aircraft lands.

- Safe procedures during landing and takeoff include the following: Remain 100 to 200 feet from the landing zone; do not allow ground personnel to approach the aircraft unless signaled to do so by an air crew member; use minimal personnel to approach the aircraft; secure loose objects that might be blown into the engine by the rotor wash; approach the aircraft from the front; stay low; and never approach the rear of the aircraft.

## ■ Follow-Up

### *Assignment follow-up from previous class:*

- What problems, if any, did you have with your assignment?
- What questions do you have?

### *In-class activities and discussion questions:*

- Discuss the rationale for safe actions when on the scene of a vehicle collision on a roadway.
- Ask students to describe legal consequences that a paramedic might encounter if involved in a collision that injures or kills someone.

### *Summary assessment:*

- Administer the quiz related to this lesson (Evolve resources, instructor's test bank).

## ■ STUDY GUIDE ANSWERS

### EXERCISE 1 ■ *Case 5: 40-year-old male—vomiting blood*

1. Does this call meet the general requirements for air medical transport? Explain your answer.

   **The driver indicated that the scene was at least 30 minutes from the closest hospital, and the paramedics are presented with a critical patient with altered level of consciousness; thus this patient may meet the requirements for air medical transport.**

2. Are there specific requirements for air medical transport in your local region that you would take into consideration on this call?

   **Local protocols will vary.**

3. Can you identify a suitable landing zone, based on what you saw in the video?

   **The lot behind the incident appears to be at least 100 × 100 feet, and no hazards are apparent; therefore the area appears to be a suitable landing zone.**

4. What additional resources might be needed to set up the landing zone?

**If police are trained, they can set up the landing zone and secure the perimeter. If they are not, you may need to request fire or rescue crews to assist with this function.**

5. When you examine the site you selected and if time is available, what measure should be taken to make the landing zone safer?

**If the fire department responds to help set up the landing zone, they may need to spray a fine mist over the area to reduce the amount of dust and debris that will be thrown by the rotor wash.**

6. If the air ambulance is not available, should you transport the patient with or without lights and sirens? Explain your answer.

**If this patient is deemed to be unstable, then transport with lights and sirens as long as this decision is consistent with local protocols.**

7. Describe how you will proceed through intersections.

**Stop at controlled intersections when going against the traffic warning devices. Make eye contact with drivers in the oncoming lane to ensure that they acknowledge your intent to proceed into the intersection. Alert other drivers by changing the tone of the siren (often to a yelp) to catch their attention. If traffic signal preempting devices are available, use them to change the signal in your favor as you travel to the hospital.**

8. What are the laws in your state as they apply to ambulance operations in emergency mode?

**Laws will vary by individual state.**

# Rescue Awareness and Operations

## ■ Assignment

### Prerequisites:

- Complete Chapter 51, Rescue Awareness and Operations, in *Mosby's Paramedic Textbook, Revised Third Edition*.
- Complete Chapter 51 in the workbook for *Mosby's Paramedic Textbook, Revised Third Edition*.
- Complete any skills or laboratory studies pertinent to this chapter.
- Read the "Getting Started" and "Orientation to Virtual Patient Encounters" sections in the *Virtual Patient Encounters Study Guide* (if this is the first lesson being attempted).

### Student assignment:

- Complete Lesson 46 in the *Virtual Patient Encounters Study Guide* after you have reviewed the topic in class.

## ■ Topic Review

### Objectives:

*On completion of this lesson, the student will be able to perform the following:*
- Identify specialized resources needed for rescue on a hazardous terrain.
- Discuss techniques to conduct a rescue on a hazardous terrain.

### Review the following topics with your students before they complete the lesson:

- Rescue requires specialized knowledge that involves both medical and mechanical skills. Paramedics must have a fundamental knowledge of rescue techniques to maintain a safe environment for themselves and their patients.
- Rescue must be a coordinated, patient-centered effort that includes accessing the patient for assessment, initiating treatment, releasing the patient, and providing continuous medical care.
- A specialized team performs most rescues in this country. Fire service or other personnel with specialized training often perform extrication and rescue. In some systems, paramedics may be cross-trained in selected rescue techniques.
- Paramedics on the rescue scene should recognize hazards associated with various environments, know when it is safe to gain access or attempt rescue, understand rescue techniques, and be skilled in patient packaging techniques needed for safe extrication.
- The priorities for safety on a rescue scene are personal safety, crew safety, bystander safety, and then rescue of the patient.

- A rescue operation has seven phases: (1) arrival and scene size-up, (2) hazard control, (3) gaining access to the patient, (4) medical treatment, (5) disentanglement, (6) patient packaging, and (7) transportation.

- Appropriate personal protective equipment should be available and worn on relevant rescue situations, including protective helmet with ear protection and chin strap, safety goggles, puncture-resistant turn-out coat, waterproof gloves, boots with steel insoles and steel toes, and self-contained breathing apparatus.

- Hazardous terrain can create difficulties during rescue operations. Hazardous terrain is classified as high-angle, low-angle, and flat terrain with obstructions.

- High-angle (vertical) rescue requires specialty training in rope rescue and aerial apparatus. Errors can result in falls that can lead to serious injury or death.

## ■ Follow-Up

### Assignment follow-up from previous class:

- What problems, if any, did you have with your assignment?
- What questions do you have?

### In-class activities and discussion questions:

- What are the possible consequences of trying to make a rescue without the proper training or equipment?
- Ask the class if anyone has been on a call during which a specialized rescue was needed. Ask the students to discuss what resources were required, what role the EMS providers played, and how long the call took.

### Summary assessment:

- Administer the quiz related to this lesson (Evolve resources, instructor's test bank).

## ■ STUDY GUIDE ANSWERS

### EXERCISE 1 ■ Case 8: 38-year-old male—suicide attempt

1. Assume that this patient jumped and was injured in his fall off the cliff. What additional resources would you need to call?

   **Call for specific fire or rescue units to assist in the extrication of the patient.**

2. What type of rescue would be involved to get him up the cliff if no access is provided from the bottom?

   **From the scene shown, high-angle rescue would apparently be needed to pull the patient up from the bottom of the hill. Then, low-angle rescue would be needed to get him from the top of the cliff and up the incline to the ambulance.**

3. What specific resource would be called in your local area?

   **Local resources will vary.**

4. What type of specialized equipment might be needed to get the patient up from the bottom of the cliff?

**Some possible equipment needed to move him up the cliff would include ropes, carabineers, pulleys, anchor points at the top of the hill, basket stretcher with restraints, long spine board, cervical collar, straps, and appropriate personal protective equipment for rescuers (gloves, harness, and helmets).**

5. Should you immediately go to care for the patient at the bottom of the cliff?

**You should go to the patient only if safe access is available. If safe access is not available, then you will need to wait until the rescue squad arrives.**

6. If you are able to access the patient to evaluate and treat him at the bottom of the cliff, what special considerations might you need to take into account?

**If you go to care for the patient, you may be able to take only a limited amount of equipment with you. Some of the equipment may be sent down in the basket stretcher. You will have to anticipate your needs before descending to where the patient is located.**

# Crime Scene Awareness

## ■ Assignment

### Prerequisites:

- Complete Chapter 52, Crime Scene Awareness, in *Mosby's Paramedic Textbook, Revised Third Edition*.
- Complete Chapter 52 in the workbook for *Mosby's Paramedic Textbook, Revised Third Edition*.
- Complete any skills or laboratory studies pertinent to this chapter.
- Read the "Getting Started" and "Orientation to Virtual Patient Encounters" sections in the *Virtual Patient Encounters Study Guide* (if this is the first lesson being attempted).

### Student assignment:

- Complete Lesson 47 in the *Virtual Patient Encounters Study Guide* after you have reviewed the topic in class.

## ■ Topic Review

### Objectives:

*On completion of this lesson, the student will be able to perform the following:*
- Identify paramedic practices to promote safety on a crime scene.
- Distinguish between cover and concealment.

### Review the following topics with your students before they complete the lesson:

- Violence against emergency medical services (EMS) providers is on the rise. Personal safety and crime scene awareness should be a top priority.
- Safety is part of the scene size-up. Unsafe scenes include large crowds, people under the influence of alcohol or drugs, on-scene violence, and known or suspected weapons.
- If you believe that the scene is unsafe, ask for law enforcement to respond. Per your agency protocol and the nature of the situation, stage at a safe distance until advised by dispatch that the scene is safe. Be on guard for deterioration of scene safety.
- Residential calls that may be dangerous include known history of violence, drug or gang area, loud noises, witnessing acts of violence, alcohol or drug use, chemical hazards, dangerous pets, and unusual darkness or silence.
- Approach a suspicious residence cautiously. Take alternate pathways to the door; do not stand in front of the ambulance lights; listen for sounds of danger; and stand to the doorknob side of the door. If evidence of danger exists, retreat and request law enforcement assistance.

- Safety tactics in dangerous situations include avoidance, tactical retreat, cover and concealment, distraction, and evasive maneuvers.
- Avoidance is the safest measure to decrease the risk of injury related to violence. Staging is an example of this technique. Tactical retreat involves immediate and rapid retreat from the scene when immediate danger is perceived.
- Cover and concealment help prevent injury. Cover behind large heavy structures provides protection from firearms. Concealment is designed to hide the rescuers but does not provide ballistic protection.

# Follow-Up

### Assignment follow-up from previous class:

- What problems, if any, did you have with your assignment?
- What questions do you have?

### In-class activities and discussion questions:

- Hide fake weapons on yourself before you teach this lesson and pull them out as you discuss this topic to show the class how easy it is to conceal a weapon. (Get appropriate clearance from security at your institution in advance, if necessary.)
- Discuss the need to ask patients about weapons (check local policies related to this).

### Summary assessment:

- Administer the quiz related to this lesson (Evolve resources, instructor's test bank).

# STUDY GUIDE ANSWERS

### EXERCISE 1 ■ *Case 11: 32-year-old male—gunshot wounds*

1. Describe where you should stage the ambulance on this call if a concern exists regarding scene safety.

   **The ambulance should be staged a safe distance from the house and within several blocks in a location where the crew is concealed from view of the scene.**

2. Look around the environment.

   a. Where would you run to seek cover?

   **Behind the adjacent structure or behind the engine block or wheel wells of the ambulance**

   b. Where would you go for concealment?

   **Behind cars or trucks**

### EXERCISE 2 ■ *Case 14: 65-year-old male—difficulty breathing*

3. Would the approach to the door by the emergency medical services (EMS) crew be acceptable if this scene were considered unsafe? Explain your answer.

   **No. The crew is positioned directly in front of the door, which is unsafe. They should approach from the side of the door if any risk of an unsafe scene exists.**

4. If you needed to retreat suddenly outside the house because a dangerous person with a gun was pursuing you, where would you seek?

   a. Concealment:

     **Behind the trees**

   b. Cover:

     **Behind the dumpster, behind the wheel wells or engine block of the ambulance, behind the adjacent structure**

# SEQUENCE OF RECOMMENDED CARE FOR VIRTUAL PATIENT ENCOUNTERS CASES

## CASE 1: 20-YEAR-OLD MALE—DIFFICULTY BREATHING (175 LB)

| RECOMMENDED INTERVENTIONS | OTHER OPTIONS | RATIONALE |
|---|---|---|
| 1. **Administer oxygen:** Apply nonrebreather mask @ 15 L/min | Nonrebreather mask @ 10-14 L/min | To provide high-concentration oxygen |
| 2. **Perform intravenous (IV) therapy:** Start left peripheral IV using normal saline or lactated Ringer's solution wide open, 500 ml | Right peripheral IV using normal saline or lactated Ringer's solution wide open, 500 ml | To provide fluid replacement and medication route |
| 3. **Administer medication:** Albuterol 2.5 mg nebulized | Albuterol 1-2 inhalations meter-dose inhaler (MDI) | To provide bronchodilation and to increase oxygen exchange |
| 4. **Administer medication:** Diphenhydramine 50 mg IV | | To block histamine |
| 5. **Administer medication:** Albuterol 2.5 mg nebulized | Albuterol 1-2 inhalations MDI | To provide bronchodilation and to increase oxygen exchange |
| 6. **Perform IV therapy:** Additional normal saline or lactated Ringer's solution, 500 ml | | To enhance perfusion by increasing blood volume |
| 7. **Administer medication:** Methylprednisolone 125 mg IV | | To provide antiinflammatory effect |
| 8. **Perform IV therapy:** Additional normal saline or lactated Ringer's solution, 500 ml | | To enhance perfusion by increasing blood volume |
| 9. **Administer medication:** Dopamine 560 mcg/min IV | Norepinephrine 7.0 mcg/min IV | Vasopressor causes vasoconstriction and increases cardiac output |
| 10. **Unload patient** | | Arrival at receiving facility |

## CASE 2: 56-YEAR-OLD FEMALE—FELL (440 LB)

| RECOMMENDED INTERVENTIONS | OTHER OPTIONS | RATIONALE |
|---|---|---|
| 1. **Administer oxygen:** Apply nonrebreather mask at 15 L/min | Nonrebreather mask at 10-14 L/min | To provide high-concentration oxygen |
| 2. **Perform IV therapy:** Start left peripheral IV using normal saline or lactated Ringer's solution to keep open (TKO) | Start right peripheral IV using normal saline or lactated Ringer's solution TKO | To provide fluid replacement and medication route |
| —PATIENT GOES INTO CARDIAC ARREST HERE— | | |
| 3. **Start cardiopulmonary resuscitation (CPR)** | | To provide perfusion |
| 4. **Remove nonrebreather mask** | | To open the airway and to assist ventilation |
| 5. **Perform airway maneuvers:** Head-tilt chin-lift | | To open airway |
| 6. **Apply airway device:** Insert oropharyngeal airway | | To maintain open airway |
| 7. **Administer oxygen:** Apply bag-mask 12 breaths @ 15 L/min | | To oxygenate and to assist ventilation |
| 8. **Remove bag-mask** | | For safety during defibrillation |
| 9. **Stop CPR** | | For safety during defibrillation |
| 10. **Apply defibrillator:** Administer 360 J unsync shock | | To convert cardiac rhythm |
| 11. **Start CPR** | | To perfuse the body's vital organs |
| 12. **Remove oropharyngeal airway** | | To allow for endotracheal intubation |
| 13. **Apply airway device:** Insert endotracheal tube | | To secure the airway |
| 14. **Administer oxygen:** Apply bag-mask 12 breaths @ 15 L/min | | To oxygenate and assist ventilation |
| 15. **Administer medication:** Epinephrine 1 mg 1:10000 IV | Vasopressin 40 U IV | To increase coronary and cerebral perfusion |
| 16. **Remove bag-mask** | | For safety during defibrillation |
| 17. **Stop CPR** | | For safety during defibrillation |
| 18. **Defibrillate:** Administer 360 J unsync shock | | To convert cardiac rhythm |
| 19. **Start CPR** | | To perfuse the body's vital organs |
| 20. **Administer oxygen:** Apply bag-mask 12 breaths @ 15 L/min | | To oxygenate and assist ventilation |

## CASE 2: 56-YEAR-OLD FEMALE—FELL (440 LB)—cont'd

| RECOMMENDED INTERVENTIONS | OTHER OPTIONS | RATIONALE |
|---|---|---|
| 21. **Administer medication:** Amiodarone 300 mg IV | Lidocaine 300 mg | May improve response to defibrillation |
| 22. **Remove bag-mask** | | For safety during defibrillation |
| 23. **Stop CPR** | | For safety during defibrillation |
| 24. **Defibrillate:** Administer 360 J unsync shock | | To convert cardiac rhythm |
| 25. **Start CPR** | | To perfuse the body's vital organs |
| 26. **Administer oxygen:** Apply bag-mask 12 breaths @ 15 L/min | | To oxygenate and assist ventilation |
| 27. **Administer medication:** Epinephrine 1 mg 1:10000 IV | Vasopressin 40 U | To increase coronary and cerebral perfusion |
| 28. **Remove bag-mask** | | For safety during defibrillation |
| 29. **Stop CPR** | | For safety during defibrillation |
| 30. **Defibrillate:** Administer 360 J unsync shock | | To convert cardiac rhythm |
| 31. **Start CPR** | | To perfuse the body's vital organs |
| 32. **Administer oxygen:** Apply bag-mask 12 breaths @ 15 L/min | | To oxygenate and assist ventilation |
| 33. **Administer medication:** Amiodarone 150 mg IV | Lidocaine 150 mg | May improve response to defibrillation |
| 34. **Remove bag-mask** | | For safety during defibrillation |
| 35. **Stop CPR** | | For safety during defibrillation |
| 36. **Defibrillate:** Administer 360 J unsync shock | | To convert cardiac rhythm |
| 37. **Start CPR** | | To perfuse the body's vital organs |
| 38. **Administer oxygen:** Apply bag-mask 12 breaths @ 15 L/min | | To oxygenate and assist ventilation |
| 39. **Administer medication:** Epinephrine 1 mg 1:10000 IV | | To increase coronary and cerebral perfusion |
| 40. **Remove bag-mask** | | For safety during defibrillation |
| 41. **Stop CPR** | | For safety during defibrillation |
| 42. **Defibrillate:** Administer 360 J unsync shock | | To convert cardiac rhythm |
| 43. **Start CPR** | | To perfuse the body's vital organs |
| 44. **Administer oxygen:** Apply bag-mask 12 breaths @ 15 L/min | | To oxygenate and assist ventilation |

## CASE 2: 56-YEAR-OLD FEMALE—FELL (440 LB)—cont'd

| RECOMMENDED INTERVENTIONS | OTHER OPTIONS | RATIONALE |
|---|---|---|
| 45. **Administer medication:** Epinephrine 1 mg 1:10000 IV | | To increase coronary and cerebral perfusion |
| 46. **Remove bag-mask** | | For safety during defibrillation |
| 47. **Stop CPR** | | For safety during defibrillation |
| 48. **Defibrillate:** Administer 360 J unsync shock | | To convert cardiac rhythm |
| —PATIENT'S RHYTHM SHOULD CONVERT TO THIRD-DEGREE HEART BLOCK HERE— | | |
| 49. **Administer oxygen:** Apply bag-mask 12 breaths @ 15 L/min | | To oxygenate and assist ventilation |
| 50. **Start pacemaker** | | To increase heart rate and perfusion |
| 51. **Administer medication:** Dopamine 1600 mcg/min | | To improve perfusion |
| 52. **Unload patient** | | Arrival at receiving facility |

## CASE 3: 7-YEAR-OLD FEMALE—SEIZURE (48 LB)

| RECOMMENDED INTERVENTIONS | OTHER OPTIONS | RATIONALE |
|---|---|---|
| 1. **Start suction** | | To clear airway |
| 2. **Stop suction** | | Airway cleared |
| 3. **Administer oxygen:** Apply nonrebreather mask @ 15 L/min | Nonrebreather mask at 12-14 L/min | To provide high-concentration oxygen |
| 4. **Perform IV therapy:** Start left peripheral IV using normal saline or lactated Ringer's solution TKO | Start right peripheral IV using normal saline or lactated Ringer's solution TKO | To provide fluid replacement and medication route |
| 5. **Administer medication:** Diazepam 1 mg IV | Lorazepam 2.5 mg IV or Midazolam 2 mg IV | To stop seizure activity |
| —BLOODY SALIVA APPEARS IN PATIENT'S MOUTH— | | |
| 6. **Remove nonrebreather mask** | | To access airway |
| 7. **Start suction** | | To clear airway |
| 8. **Stop suction** | | Airway cleared |
| 9. **Apply airway device:** Insert oropharyngeal airway | Nasopharyngeal airway | To maintain open airway |
| 10. **Administer oxygen:** Apply bag-mask 20 breaths @ 15 L/min | 20 breaths @ 14 L/min 12 breaths @ 14 L/min 12 breaths @ 15 L/min | To ventilate and provide supplemental oxygen |
| 11. **Perform IV therapy:** Additional normal saline or lactated Ringer's solution, 500 ml | 250 ml | To enhance perfusion by increasing blood volume |
| 12. **Unload patient** | | Arrival at receiving facility |

## CASE 4: 64-YEAR-OLD MALE—UNKNOWN MEDICAL (155 LB)

| RECOMMENDED INTERVENTIONS | OTHER OPTIONS | RATIONALE |
| --- | --- | --- |
| 1. **Administer oxygen:** Apply nasal cannula 6 L/min | Nasal cannula 1-5 L/min | To provide supplemental oxygen |
| 2. **Administer medication:** Glucagon 1 mg intramuscular (IM) | Oral glucose 15 g | To increase blood glucose |
| 3. **Administer medication:** Glucagon 1 mg IM | Oral glucose 15 g | To increase blood glucose |
| 4. **Unload patient** | | Arrival at receiving facility |

## CASE 5: 40-YEAR-OLD MALE—VOMITING BLOOD (186 LB)

| RECOMMENDED INTERVENTIONS | OTHER OPTIONS | RATIONALE |
|---|---|---|
| 1. **Administer oxygen:** Apply nonrebreather mask @ 15 L/min | Nonrebreather mask @ 12-14 L/min or bag-mask @ 15 L/min | To provide high-concentration oxygen (and to assist ventilation if bag-mask is used) |
| 2. **Perform IV therapy:** Start left peripheral IV using normal saline or lactated Ringer's solution, 500 ml wide open | Start right peripheral IV using normal saline or lactated Ringer's solution, 500 ml wide open | To provide fluid resuscitation |
| 3. **Perform IV therapy:** Start right peripheral IV using normal saline or lactated Ringer's solution, 500 ml wide open | Start left peripheral IV using normal saline or lactated Ringer's solution, 500 ml wide open | To provide fluid resuscitation |
| 4. **Perform IV therapy:** Additional normal saline or lactated Ringer's solution to left or right peripheral, 500 ml wide open | | To provide fluid resuscitation |
| —PATIENT VOMITS HERE— | | |
| 5. **Remove oxygen device** | | To prepare to suction |
| 6. **Start suction** | | To remove bloody vomitus |
| 7. **Stop suction** | | Airway cleared |
| 8. **Administer oxygen:** Apply nonrebreather mask @ 15 L/min | Nonrebreather mask @ 12-14 L/min or bag-mask @ 15 L/min | To provide high-concentration oxygen (and assist ventilation if bag-mask is used) |
| 9. **Perform IV therapy:** Additional normal saline or lactated Ringer's solution to left or right peripheral, 500 ml wide open | | To provide fluid resuscitation |
| 10. **Unload patient** | | Arrival at receiving facility |

## CASE 6: 16-YEAR-OLD FEMALE—UNKNOWN MEDICAL (88 LB)

| RECOMMENDED INTERVENTIONS | OTHER OPTIONS | RATIONALE |
|---|---|---|
| 1. **Perform airway maneuver:** Head-tilt chin-lift | Jaw thrust | To open airway |
| 2. **Start suction** | | To clear airway |
| 3. **Stop suction** | | Airway cleared |
| 4. **Apply airway device:** Insert nasopharyngeal airway | | To maintain open airway |
| 5. **Administer oxygen:** Apply bag-mask 12 breaths @ 15 L/min | Bag-mask 12 breaths @ 14 L/min or nonrebreather mask @ 12-15 L/min | To provide high-concentration oxygen (and assist ventilation if bag-mask is used) |
| 6. **Perform IV therapy:** Start left peripheral IV using normal saline or lactated Ringer's solution, 500 ml wide open | Right peripheral IV, 500 ml wide open or left or right peripheral IV, 250 ml wide open | To provide fluid replacement and medication route |
| —PATIENT BEGINS TO EXHIBIT SEIZURE ACTIVITY— | | |
| 7. **Administer medication:** Diazepam 5 mg IV | Lorazepam 4 mg IV | To stop seizure activity |
| 8. **Remove oxygen administration device** | | To access airway |
| 9. **Start suction** | | To clear airway |
| 10. **Stop suction** | | Airway cleared |
| 11. **Administer oxygen:** Apply bag-mask 12 breaths @ 15 L/min | Bag-mask 12 breaths @ 14 L/min or nonrebreather mask @ 12-15 L/min | To provide high-concentration oxygen (and assist ventilation if bag-mask is used) |
| 12. **Administer medication:** Sodium bicarbonate 50 mEq IV | | To reverse cardiac toxicity from tricyclic antidepressants (TCAs) |
| 13. **Perform IV therapy:** Additional normal saline or lactated Ringer's solution, 500 ml wide open | Additional normal saline or lactated Ringer's solution, 250 ml wide open | To enhance perfusion |
| 14. **Unload patient** | | Arrival at receiving facility |

## CASE 7: 8-YEAR-OLD MALE—SUBMERSION (66 LB)

| RECOMMENDED INTERVENTIONS | OTHER OPTIONS | RATIONALE |
| --- | --- | --- |
| 1. **Apply cervical collar** | Open airway with jaw thrust maneuver | To provide spinal stabilization |
| 2. **Perform airway maneuver:** Jaw thrust | If airway maneuver performed already, apply cervical collar | To open airway |
| 3. **Start suction** | | To clear airway |
| 4. **Stop suction** | | To clear airway |
| 5. **Administer oxygen:** Apply bag-mask 12 breaths @ 15 L/min | | To oxygenate and assist ventilation |
| 6. **Remove bag-mask** | | To prepare for intubation |
| 7. **Apply airway device:** Insert endotracheal tube | | To maintain open airway |
| 8. **Administer oxygen:** Apply bag-mask 12 breaths @ 15 L/min | | To oxygenate and assist ventilation |
| —FLUID REAPPEARS IN PATIENT'S AIRWAY— | | |
| 9. **Remove bag-mask** | | To prepare to suction |
| 10. **Start suction** | | To clear airway |
| 11. **Stop suction** | | Airway cleared |
| 12. **Administer oxygen:** Apply bag-mask 12 breaths @ 15 L/min | | To oxygenate and assist ventilation |
| 13. **Apply long backboard** | | To provide spinal stabilization |
| 14. **Apply dressings** | | To control bleeding |
| 15. **Perform IV therapy:** Start left peripheral IV using normal saline or lactated Ringer's solution TKO | Start right peripheral IV using normal saline or lactated Ringer's solution TKO | To provide medication route |
| 16. **Unload patient** | | Arrival at receiving facility |

### CASE 8: 38-YEAR-OLD MALE—SUICIDE ATTEMPT (196 LB)

| RECOMMENDED INTERVENTIONS | OTHER OPTIONS | RATIONALE |
|---|---|---|
| 1. **Perform IV therapy:** Start left peripheral IV using normal saline or lactated Ringer's solution TKO | Start right peripheral IV using normal saline or lactated Ringer's solution TKO | To provide fluid replacement and medication route |
| 2. **Administer medication:** Midazolam 2 mg IV | Diazepam 5 or 10 mg IV; Halperidol 5 mg IM; or Lorazepam 2-4 mg IV or IM | To provide sedation |
| 3. **Administer oxygen:** Apply nonrebreather mask @ 15 L/min | Nasal cannula @ 4-6 L/min; Simple face mask @ 6-10 L/min; Partial rebreather mask @ 6-10 L/min; or Nonrebreather mask @ 10-14 L/min | To provide supplemental oxygen |
| —PATIENT BECOMES ALERT AND COMBATIVE WHEN LOADED INTO AMBULANCE— | | |
| 4. **Administer medication:** Midazolam 2 mg IV | Diazepam 5 or 10 mg IV; Halperidol 5 mg IM; or Lorazepam 2-4 mg IV or IM | To provide sedation |
| 5. **Unload patient** | | Arrival at receiving facility |

## CASE 9: 22-YEAR-OLD FEMALE—ASSAULT (142 LB)

| RECOMMENDED INTERVENTIONS | OTHER OPTIONS | RATIONALE |
|---|---|---|
| 1. **Administer oxygen:** Apply nonrebreather mask @ 15 L/min | Nasal cannula 1-6 L/min; Simple face mask 6-10 L/min; Partial rebreather mask 6-10 L/min; or Nonrebreather mask 10-14 L/min | To provide supplemental oxygen |
| 2. **Apply cervical collar** | | To stabilize cervical spine |
| 3. **Apply long backboard** | | To immobilize cervical spine |
| 4. **Perform IV therapy:** Start peripheral IV using normal saline or lactated Ringer's solution wide open (250 or 500 ml) or TKO **Apply dressings** | **NOTE:** These two interventions (IV therapy in either left or right peripheral and apply dressings) can be performed in any order | To support perfusion and provide medication route<br><br>To control bleeding |
| 5. **Administer medication:** Morphine sulfate 2 or 4 mg IV | Fentanyl 100 mcg IV; Meperidine 20 or 35 mg IV; Meperidine 50 or 100 mg IM; or Nitrous oxide:oxygen | To relieve pain |
| 6. **Administer medication:** Morphine sulfate 2 or 4 mg IV | Fentanyl 100 mcg IV; Meperidine 20 or 35 mg IV; Meperidine 50 or 100 mg IM; or Nitrous oxide:oxygen | To relieve pain |
| 7. **Unload patient** | | Arrival at receiving facility |

## CASE 10: 25-YEAR-OLD FEMALE—ABDOMINAL PAIN (186 LB)

| RECOMMENDED INTERVENTIONS | OTHER OPTIONS | RATIONALE |
|---|---|---|
| 1. **Administer oxygen:** Apply nonrebreather mask @ 15 L/min | Nonrebreather mask @ 12-14 L/min | To provide high-concentration oxygen |
| 2. **Perform IV therapy:** Start left peripheral IV using normal saline or lactated Ringer's solution TKO | Start right peripheral IV using normal saline or lactated Ringer's solution TKO | To provide fluid replacement and medication route |
| 3. **Administer medication:** Magnesium sulfate 2 g IV | | To prevent seizure activity and inhibit uterine contractions |
| 4. **Unload patient** | | Arrival at receiving facility |

## CASE 11: 32-YEAR-OLD MALE—GUNSHOT WOUNDS (220 LB)

| RECOMMENDED INTERVENTIONS | OTHER OPTIONS | RATIONALE |
|---|---|---|
| 1. **Perform airway maneuvers**: Jaw thrust | **NOTE:** Interventions 1, 2, and 4 may be interchanged to allow flexibility to follow local protocols. | To open airway |
| 2. **Apply airway devices:** Insert oropharyngeal airway | | To maintain open airway |
| 3. **Administer oxygen:** Apply bag-mask 12 breaths @ 15 L/min | | To provide high-concentration oxygen and ventilate |
| 4. **Apply cervical collar** | | To provide spinal stabilization |
| 5. **Perform needle decompression** | | To relieve tension pneumothorax |
| 6. **Remove bag-mask** | | To prepare for endotracheal intubation |
| 7. **Remove oropharyngeal airway** | | To prepare for endotracheal intubation |
| 8. **Apply airway devices:** Insert endotracheal tube | | To secure the airway |
| 9. **Administer oxygen:** Apply bag-mask 12 breaths @ 15 L/min | | To provide supplemental oxygen and ventilate |
| 10. **Apply dressings** | **NOTE:** Interventions 10 and 11 may occur anytime during this case to allow flexibility to follow local protocols. | To control bleeding |
| 11. **Apply long backboard** | | To provide spinal stabilization |
| 12. **Perform IV therapy:** Start left peripheral IV using normal saline or lactated Ringer's solution, 500 ml wide open | Start right peripheral IV using normal saline or lactated Ringer's solution, 500 ml wide open | To enhance perfusion by increasing blood volume |
| 13. **Perform IV therapy:** Start right peripheral IV using normal saline or lactated Ringer's solution, 500 ml wide open | Start left peripheral IV using normal saline or lactated Ringer's solution, 500 ml wide open | To enhance perfusion by increasing blood volume |
| 14. **Unload patient** | | Arrival at receiving facility |

## CASE 12: 57-YEAR-OLD MALE—MAN DOWN (220 LB)

| RECOMMENDED INTERVENTIONS | OTHER OPTIONS | RATIONALE |
|---|---|---|
| 1. **Administer oxygen:** Apply nonrebreather mask @ 15 L/min | Nonrebreather mask @ 12-14 L/min | To provide supplemental oxygen |
| 2. **Load patient** | | To provide transport to definitive care |
| 3. **Perform IV therapy:** Start left peripheral IV using normal saline or lactated Ringer's solution, 500 ml wide open | Start right peripheral IV using Ringer's solution, 500 ml wide open | To provide fluid replacement and medication route |
| 4. **Perform IV therapy:** Start right peripheral IV using normal saline or lactated Ringer's solution, 500 ml wide open | Start left peripheral IV using Ringer's solution, 500 ml wide open | To provide fluid replacement and medication route |
| 5. **Unload patient** | | Arrival at receiving facility |

## CASE 13: 5-MONTH-OLD MALE—UNRESPONSIVE (16 LB)

| RECOMMENDED INTERVENTIONS | OTHER OPTIONS | RATIONALE |
| --- | --- | --- |
| 1. **Perform airway maneuver:** Head-tilt/chin-lift | | To open the airway |
| 2. **Start suction** | | To clear airway |
| 3. **Stop suction** | | Airway cleared |
| 4. **Start CPR** | | To provide perfusion |
| 5. **Apply airway devices:** Insert oropharyngeal airway | | To open the airway |
| 6. **Administer oxygen:** Apply bag-mask 20 breaths @ 15 L/min | Bag-mask 20 breaths @ 14 L/min or Bag-mask 12 breaths @ 14-15 L/min | To provide high-concentration oxygen and assist ventilation |
| 7. **Remove bag-mask** | | For safety during defibrillation |
| 8. **Stop CPR** | | For safety during defibrillation |
| 9. **Defibrillate:** Administer 15 J unsync shock | | To convert cardiac rhythm |
| 10. **Start CPR** | Beginning with chest compressions | To provide perfusion |
| 11. **Remove oropharyngeal airway** | | To insert endotracheal tube |
| 12. **Apply airway devices:** Insert endotracheal tube | | To secure the airway |
| 13. **Administer oxygen:** Apply bag-mask 20 breaths @ 15 L/min | Bag-mask 20 breaths @ 14 L/min or Bag-mask 12 breaths @ 14-15 L/min | To provide high-concentration oxygen and assist ventilation |
| 14. **Perform IV therapy:** Establish intraosseous access using normal saline or lactated Ringer's solution TKO | Establish intraosseous access using dextrose 5% water ($D_5W$) TKO | To provide fluid replacement and medication route |
| 15. **Administer medication:** Epinephrine 0.075 mg 1:10000 IO | | To increase coronary and cerebral perfusion |
| 16. **Remove bag-mask** | | For safety during defibrillation |
| 17. **Stop CPR** | | For safety during defibrillation |
| 18. **Defibrillate:** Administer 25 J unsync shock | | To convert cardiac rhythm |
| —PATIENT'S ECG RHYTHM CONVERTS TO SINUS BRADYCARDIA— | | |
| 19. **Administer oxygen:** Apply bag-mask 20 breaths @ 15 L/min | Bag-mask 20 breaths @ 14 L/min or Bag-mask 12 breaths @ 14-15 L/min | To provide high-concentration oxygen and assist ventilation |
| 20. **Unload patient** | | Arrival at receiving facility |

## CASE 14: 65-YEAR-OLD MALE—DIFFICULTY BREATHING (198 LB)

| RECOMMENDED INTERVENTIONS | OTHER OPTIONS | RATIONALE |
|---|---|---|
| 1. **Administer oxygen:** Apply nonrebreather mask @ 15 L/min | | To provide high-concentration oxygen |
| 2. **Perform IV therapy:** Start left peripheral IV using normal saline or lactated Ringer's solution TKO | Start right peripheral IV using normal saline or lactated Ringer's solution TKO | To provide fluid replacement and medication route |
| 3. **Administer medications:** <ul><li>Nitroglycerin 0.4 mg SL</li><li>Furosemide 40 mg IV</li><li>Morphine Sulfate 4 mg IV</li></ul> | **NOTE:** These three medications can be administered in any order. | • To decrease workload of the heart<br>• To reduce cardiac preload and lung congestion<br>• To decrease myocardial oxygen demand |
| 4. **Unload patient** | | Arrival at receiving facility |

## CASE 15: 42-YEAR-OLD MALE—DIFFICULTY BREATHING (165 LB)

| RECOMMENDED INTERVENTIONS | OTHER OPTIONS | RATIONALE |
| --- | --- | --- |
| 1. **Administer oxygen:** Apply nonrebreather mask @ 15 L/min | Nonrebreather mask @ 12-14 L/min | To provide high-concentration oxygen |
| 2. **Perform IV therapy:** Start left peripheral IV using normal saline or lactated Ringer's solution TKO | Start right peripheral IV using normal saline or lactated Ringer's solution TKO | To provide fluid replacement and medication route |
| 3. **Load patient** | | To provide transport to definitive care |
| 4. **Unload patient** | | Arrival at receiving facility |